Our Fractured Wholeness

Our Fractured Wholeness

*Making the Courageous Journey
from Brokenness to Love*

Diana Ventura

CASCADE *Books* · Eugene, Oregon

OUR FRACTURED WHOLENESS
Making the Courageous Journey from Brokenness to Love

Cascade Books
An Imprint of Wipf and Stock Publishers
199 W. 8th Ave., Suite 3
Eugene, OR 97401

www.wipfandstock.com

ISBN 13: 978-1-60899-009-2

Cataloging-in-Publication data:

Ventura, Diana.

Our fractured wholeness : making the courageous journey from brokenness to
love / Diana Ventura.

x + 114 p. ; 23 cm.

ISBN 13: 978-1-60899-009-2

1. Spiritual life. 2. Suffering. 3. People with disabilities—Religious aspects—
Christianity. 4. Healing and Christianity. I. Title.

BT732.7 V41 2010

Manufactured in the U.S.A.

*For God and all those whose love and support
helped to nurture this book into being, especially*

Margaret A. Hothem

Cindy Keefe

Elizabeth A. Musselman

Stephanie Paulsell

Leslie E. Sternberg

&

David Tracy

Contents

Acknowledgments

I KNOW THAT SOMEWHERE in the universe of saints my parents are smiling down upon these pages, glad that my words have finally found their way into print. To my parents, and my siblings—Mariann, Joe, Sue, Paul, Edie, Tina, and Bernie (who unfortunately is no longer with us; may he rest in peace)—I owe a great debt of gratitude. A special note of acknowledgement goes out to my extended large family filled with aunts, uncles and cousins (too many to mention here by name) who helped me on my way. Thank you, every one of you, for always holding a loving hopefulness and unwavering belief in me. Your hope and belief live in all my accomplishments and many satisfied dreams.

This book is just another one of those dreams turned into reality. I wish to thank all those who, through their dedication and encouragement, carried that same loving hope and helped this book come to fruition—readers, editors, and those who simply encouraged me along the way, especially Mary Bryant, Jan Carlberg, Sean Clark, Kris Culp, Bill and Patti Crowl, Carole Drago, Toni DeLorenzo, Mike Givens, Colleen Griffith, Priscilla Hardy, Laura Ruth Jerrett, Ayanna Johnson, Laurie Malcom, Jane McBride, Jamie Murray, Jen Nagel, Joy Omslaer, Jamie Polsen, Carol Saunders, Kathryn Tanner, Dawna Thomas, Susan Troy, Arlene Uslander, and Betsy Perry White. A special note of thanks goes to LaVonne Neff, Ulrike Gutherie, and K. C. Hanson for their fine editing and their dedicated efforts to make this book everything it was meant to be.

I dedicate this book to God. When I began writing it, I said a little prayer that went something like this: "I pray that every word, every sentence, and every page will give glory to you, Almighty God." I pray now in thanksgiving that my little prayer has been answered. I pray also that those who need to hear some echo of truth in these pages will do so, and that through what is written here God will bring new love and life into being.

God bless all my many readers.

ONE

God, Brokenness, and the Tragic Event

M Y BODY HAS A voice, and the word it speaks is love. How can my body speak such a word when my body is broken and disabled?

Years ago, I thought my body was despicable. I would say to myself, "How dare you lack beauty and strength?" Since then, I've journeyed with God through sadness, pain, and anger, and I have come to a place where I love my disabled body. To love is to say, "It is wonderful that you exist."[1]

I wish to share some of my healing journey with you in the hope that you too may say, "It is wonderful that I exist just as I am." I seek to bring you to a place where you know the meaning of your brokenness. I want to travel like an adventurer with you into the frontiers of your heart as you unravel the mystery of your brokenness and relationship with God.

To penetrate the mystery of how God meets you in your brokenness is to take a journey through your own personal jungle of hope and despair. My hope is that my story and theological reflections will help you navigate the rough terrain of your inner soul so that you may know love even in the deepest, darkest, most painful parts of your being.

Before beginning to tell my story, I must tell you some of the basic assumptions from which I am writing. I will use my personal experience with disability as a metaphor for the brokenness that we all experience. Disability is one particular form of the brokenness that comes to us all by way of tragedy. No human life is exempt from an encounter with tragedy. No one can predict the day or hour when tragedy will strike. We cannot know in advance when tragedy will come to us. The only thing we can be assured of is that tragedy and the brokenness it brings will be with us in some form or other until the end of time.

---

1. Josef Pieper, *Faith, Hope, Love* (San Francisco: Ignatius, 1997) 170.

Human violence is one way tragedy comes to us. When we think of tragedy, perhaps we recollect the ovens of Auschwitz, the dead bodies piled one upon the other, tangled up as if they were one, bodies that were once people with lives and families. Perhaps we see photographs of emaciated people in striped, tattered clothes staring back at us with desperate eyes, and we wonder how humankind can find its way into such darkness.

In this book, I will not attempt to explain why such human violence exists or how to eradicate it. My words cannot wash away the pain of Auschwitz or make sense of September 11. Rather, I will focus on how to soothe the pain of physical brokenness no matter how it comes to us. This is not to say that my words will have no meaning for the soldier who comes back from war missing a limb. I hope I can offer him or her some comfort. But I will not try to explain why the bomb was in the air, or why it landed where it did. For centuries theologians and philosophers have attempted to answer questions about why human violence and suffering exist. My efforts to answer such questions are likely only to echo the same fragmentary truth thought out in the minds of many who have come before me. So my intent here is to explore what we are to do about our suffering, rather than answer the question of why.

Physical brokenness is always an unwelcome, tragic event, no matter what its origin. An event happens, and then we are changed. We are in a car accident and lose a limb or sustain a head injury and are now limited in the way we can think and move. We are born missing fingers or toes, or with organs that do not function as they should. One minute we call ourselves healthy, and the next minute the doctor's phone call turns us into a patient with a diagnosis. Without warning we are stricken with heart attacks, strokes, cancer, diabetes, or other afflictions that leave us broken, ill, suffering, or disabled. I will be speaking of such events that arrive on our doorstep, not through human violence, but through random chance. It's the luck of the draw—a flip of the coin—and we are asked to endure.

We hang on for dear life even as we are made weak, cut off and disconnected from our previous life. Our brokenness puts a host of new obstacles in our path. It penetrates every level of our being and gives us suffering, pain, and anguish. It leaves us grief stricken and in despair because it is inescapable. Banging and clamoring for attention, our pain will not leave us alone. We know our lives will never be the same. There is no turning back, no starting over, no way to magically wipe away the events that have occurred. And it is with just this type of event that my parents and I would be asked to contend.

THE TRAGIC EVENT AT MY BIRTH

Even before I have life outside the womb, I am going to die: "Somebody, please, help me! I can't hold on to life. My mother's womb won't keep me any longer and I am coming out now."

"It isn't time to come out. You are nearly two months premature," a voice calls out of nowhere.

I reply to the strange voice, saying, "I need more time to grow."

As my journey to life continues, I think: "It's time, it's time, and I must be born now. I must have a separate being. Now, right now, I must be born. There is no more time to wait. She can't hold me any longer. I have no choice but to come out of my mother's womb and live." As my mother pushes, I hear the faint sounds of life outside her womb. But death seeks to steal my approaching life, because my body is finding no nourishment of air. I feel the doctor's hands surrounding me when my lungs begin to fail.

"Blue, blue, blue; she's turning blue!" A frantic rush begins in the delivery room to resuscitate my failing lungs. Each moment without oxygen brings with it a small measure of death. Every small death adds upon the other until lasting and final death closes in on me. It appears that death will win the battle, because life cannot withstand the lack of oxygen. I give death no heed, and yet death continues to intrude upon my desire for life. As the battle between life and death rages on in the delivery room, in my mind I travel to the center of the universe to meet my Maker.

When I reach the center of the universe, I feel God's presence surrounding me in much the same way as my mother held me in her womb. I cannot see God with my eyes, but I know the divine presence is with me because love envelops my soul. For in the very moments my fate is being decided, my soul knows only peace. In the quiet of such assuring love, I am ready to give up the fight for life and allow my soul to rest in this peace forever.

In this calm stillness, as I rest in the holiness and peace of love, God speaks to me. I hear no words, and yet I comprehend the meaning just the same. God asks, "Why are you here?"

Puzzled, I whisper, "You don't know?"

"Tell me in your own words," I hear back.

So I respond, "I am trying to be born, but death is trying to take my life. I didn't know what to do, so I thought I would come to the center of the universe to ask you, God, the creator and sustainer of all life. God, I know that in the beginning, your Holy Spirit was moving, and light became light, the heavens were the heavens, dry land was formed, day and night were born, stars established their light in the sky, and humankind found its way into being. And behold, all creation was good. I know that your spirit moving hither and yon in the universe created all that is known and all that is beyond my comprehension. And on this day, your spirit came to move precisely on everything that was necessary to create me, and the time came for me to be born. Now death seeks to take my life, and I know that you, God, are the one to ask for help."

God asks me, "What is it that you seek?"

I reply, "All I want is life. I want to know the beauty of love and happiness and all the wonder that life brings."

God continues, "So you want to live?"

"Yes, yes, I want to live," I say.

Then God speaks to me: "Let there be life for you. You are called to have life and have it abundantly. You are called to have life even though you touched the brink of death. Some are not."

I ask, "How is it that some are called to life and some are not?"

God replies, "That is a mystery not to be explained. It is only to be acknowledged and known." Then God asks me, "Do you choose life no matter what it will bring you?"

I reply, "God, I choose life. Let there be life for me no matter the consequences."

My unconditional acceptance moves God to command the universe. God says, "Let there be life for this little one," and God breathes life into me. And at God's word, death concedes defeat. In that instant, my life is restored.

∾

Death will try again to wield its power. Four days later, on Christmas Day 1964, death sneaks up on me as I lie in an incubator seeking to establish life. My lungs fail a second time. I turn not only blue, but also black. Death does not quit until it pierces me with tragedy. As the doctors and nurses rush to save me once again, my brain cells begin to die.

I find myself back at the center of the universe. I ask God, "What am I doing here again? I thought my battle with death and darkness was over."

God replies, "My child, the battle between death and life rages throughout all of life. One must be willing to commit to life regardless of the consequences."

I protest, "But God, look at my brain cells dying left and right. I certainly will be lacking. This event is a tragedy, to say the least. If everything in creation is good, why is such a tragic event happening?"

God says, "All of these questions are cloaked in mystery and are beyond ordinary human comprehension. Such understanding will require spiritual insight and a mystical vision. Your journey through life will give you clues to answer your questions, but you will find no definitive answers."

There is a pause. The time with God has left me stunned and dazed, but I manage to ask, "What will happen if I choose life now?"

God is silent for a time and then asks me again, "Diana, do you choose life no matter the consequences?"

Not knowing how or why, I reply, "Yes, God. I choose life no matter the consequences, because I can't die before I have a chance to live!"

"That's right," God says. "You can't die before you have had a chance to live. Go back! Go back, and day by day you will come to understand the meaning of your unwelcome encounter with death and tragedy. Know this, my little one—as with everyone on the face of the earth, I will always be with you. I will never leave you. I will watch over you with a loving eye and a caring hand." And then God sends me on my way to travel through life as a pilgrim, as one on a journey.

≈

When I was revived to continue my work at establishing life, no one thought further about the incident. Life went on as if it were normal. But now that I had encountered death, my life was changed. The brain cells that died during my early days would surely be missed. A lifelong battle with cerebral palsy would be my fate.

Because of cerebral palsy, my lower limbs do not work properly. My movements are awkward and jerky. My muscles are subject to spasms, which force me to move in directions I don't want to go. Suddenly I find myself diving for the floor or smashing into walls. These problems have to do with confusion in the messages sent from my brain through my nerves to my muscles. At times, these messages work like reverberating circuits, repeating over and over again. It is as if my muscles hear the message to contract a thousand times when a normal person hears it only once. As a result, my balance is completely off. A person stands a better chance of finding diamonds on a busy street than I have of standing on one foot for more than ten seconds. Nearly every day I trip and fall. All of a sudden, it happens. My foot scrapes the protruding uneven edge of a sidewalk, or it catches on something like a floor mat. A scatter rug becomes a flying carpet, and I am diving for the floor. With a quick tuck-and-roll, I protect my head and other body parts. Don't worry; after many years I've perfected the art of falling. I hardly ever get hurt.

Sometimes I do have a close call. Recently I nearly bashed my head against a cement retaining wall that is right outside my back door. My building is deserted during the day. So when my foot caught the door-jamb and my head went straight for the cement wall, I knew that if my attempt to tuck my head into my body failed, I would most surely be left bleeding for hours. My tuck worked. I missed the wall by less than an inch. As I gathered myself after the fall, rolling over on all fours, I thought, "For years, my falling has felt like an art form that I have perfected, but now I have to believe that something more is at work." I felt as if an army of angels was surrounding me and protecting me. I pushed myself up by grabbing onto the wall that had just nearly killed me. Shocked from the close call, I began whispering to myself, "It must be God who spared me. It must be God who kept me from getting hurt."

God's love seems to have kept me from harm's way that day, and yet—why does God not protect us from harm every day?

We cannot know why in one instance God seems to have spared us some terrible event, while at the next moment we are crying out, "God, why are you allowing this to happen?" Why does God not reach out with his holy hands and almighty power to prevent tragic events?

A man I know went on retreat with the Jesuits. He was trying to figure out whether to commit his life to the Society of Jesus, because he loved God and truly wanted to serve. He decided to go swimming with some children in the small Costa Rican village where he was staying. He stood on the dock and dove right in, not realizing that the water was very shallow and that rocks hid just below the surface. His head hit one of the rocks and he broke his neck. He was instantly paralyzed from the neck down.

A priest pulled him out of the water and knelt down next to him. "How could this have happened?" the man cried out.

The priest looked into his eyes and said, "Life is very fragile."

I like the priest's response, because it acknowledges the mystery of life. We can't know the definitive answer as to why we suffer, but suffer we all do.

How do we explain the tragedy and brokenness that comes into our lives through no choice of our own? God seems to have fashioned the universe in such a way that life includes death and death includes life. This is not to say that God maliciously plays with our lives. It appears that we can't have love and goodness without also having their by-products: death and tragedy. This is the reality that creates our everyday lives. New life greets us in the morning, but a measure of death approaches us at the end of the day. Every day, from the moment we are born, we are in the process of both living and dying.

Some argue that the tragedy we experience is not willed by God but is the consequence of natural laws at work within creation. For instance, the anoxia or lack of oxygen to my brain at my birth created my disability and brokenness. The natural law in this case is that brain cells require oxygen in order to live: when their oxygen supply is cut off, the only possible result is that they die. When enough brain cells die, cerebral palsy results. Natural laws can only operate in the way they were designed and cannot violate themselves to prevent disability. So physical brokenness—my disability—results from circumstances interacting with natural laws.

Others find fault with this approach, since God, being greater than nature, can create and intervene at will. We are back in the realm of mystery; there are no clear explanations for tragedy. But in spite of the persistence of natural laws that sometimes help us and sometimes hurt us, one truth is sure: God remains ready, willing, and able to relate intimately with every person in this world, for just as suffering and tragedy are part of the universe, so also is the love of God.

How can I say this? Four months after my birth, my being would find its way to God's love through baptism. Drops of water were mysteriously transformed into a love far beyond what we can manifest on our own, the love that comes only from God. As those tiny drops fell on my little forehead, the Episcopal priest said, "Diana, I baptize you in the Name of the Father, and of the Son, and of the Holy Spirit. Amen."

Then the congregation prayed: "Heavenly Father, we thank you that by water and the Holy Spirit you have bestowed upon Diana your servant the forgiveness of sin, and have raised her to the new life of grace. Sustain her, O Lord, in your Holy Spirit. Give her an inquiring and discerning heart, the courage to will and to persevere, a spirit to know and to love you, and the gift of joy and wonder in all your works. Amen."[2]

~

My life as a Christian began on that day. The prayers of the congregation would truly be answered, for throughout my life I would know the new life of grace, the Holy Spirit would sustain me, and I would be given an inquiring and discerning heart along with the courage to will and to persevere. The single act of baptism would be the foundation for my life in God. It would lead me to transformation, healing, and love.

In baptism, we are welcomed into the family of God and receive the light of Christ forever. Baptism will not remove or help us avoid tragic events. It does not promise to take away our brokenness. My cerebral palsy was not magically washed away by the waters of baptism. Instead, something different occurred: I would find love even in great difficulties. I would hear God's voice speaking through my physical difficulties. I would know God, and God would know me through all these challenges.

I am not saying that it is better for me to have cerebral palsy than to be physically whole. Of course not. I am saying that God speaks and acts mysteriously even through our brokenness. In fact nothing—not tragedy, not sickness, not disability, not even death—can separate us from the love of God. And at baptism, my intimate relationship with God would begin, where I would come to know a life in which love and tragedy are married as one.

My parents had no idea that tragedy had struck. Everyone believed I had escaped death to resume a happy, normal life. However, when I was fourteen months old and still only crawling around on my belly like a

2. *The Book of Common Prayer* (New York: Oxford University Press, 1979) 308.

soldier in the trenches, my mother knew something was wrong. She had raised five children before me, and my inability to walk or even crawl on hands and knees sent alarm bells ringing through her head. My pediatrician responded to her concerns, not by giving her even a faint hint of his suspicions, but by writing a letter to Children's Hospital in Boston saying he thought cerebral palsy was my fate. He then sent her to doctors at Children's Hospital for the verdict.

My mother often expressed anger toward that pediatrician for preparing her so poorly for what lay ahead. On their initial visit to Children's, my parents would be asked to accept unconditionally the tragic event of my complicated birth. They would be required to commit themselves to helping me create the most of my life in spite of its difficult beginning.

THE DIAGNOSIS

The doctor announced, "She won't amount to anything. She needs an institution."

Fourteen months old, I cried out and asked for my mother. There was nothing wrong with my cognition.

My father grabbed the doctor by his white lab coat, spun him around, and threw him out of the examining room. I don't remember the incident, but I can see these events because my mother has told me the story many times. In my mind's eye, I see the doctor's arms and legs flailing as my father's rage intensifies. I see my father's clenched fist pulling the doctor's lab coat close to him so that his green-gray eyes, bald head, and five-o'clock shadow get right up into the doctor's face. I can hear my father say to the doctor as he grabs him by the throat, "I may look like a working man, but I am not stupid." My mother, probably in a nervous silence, holds me, calms me down—privately pleased for my father's rage while also hoping that it will not get out of hand. My father swings the doctor around and throws him out the door.

Out in the hallway, my father grabbed another doctor by his lab coat and shoved him into the examining room. "You examine my daughter!" my father roared. The second doctor probably said to himself, "I'll say anything to save myself from this lunatic." But as he took me in his hands and moved my legs around, and as my anxious and frightened parents more calmly expressed their concerns and explained the inappropriate actions of the other doctor, he began to understand what had happened.

The second doctor concluded that my cerebral palsy was mild. I would have some problems, but for the most part I would be fine. I would not need an institution.

As my mother used to tell the story, my father put his face in his hands and cried after the second doctor left the room. "Why me twice? Why me twice?" My father's brother was born with cerebral palsy. My grandmother cared for my uncle until he was in his twenties and became too heavy for her to lift. In those days, there was nothing she could do but put him in a "special hospital" (i.e., an institution) where he could be cared for. I believe that a deep sadness and fear created my father's rage. He carried a deep sense of sorrow for his brother's fate.

Back in the twenties when my uncle was born, families didn't usually keep disabled people in their homes. Those with disabilities were more often warehoused in institutions. So my Italian grandmother, a widow with seven children, did a remarkable thing in keeping her son home for so many years. I often felt that in my father's heart, I walked in the shadow of his brother's fate, redeeming it by the full life that I would live. My father had great respect for both human and animal life: he would open the door to let a fly out of the house or would catch a spider and turn it loose in the yard. It would be impossible for him to "put me away," especially knowing how long his brother had lived with his family.

The doctor who thought I needed an institution believed that life with a disability was not worth living. He thought he had all the information he needed about my life in order to make a prediction that my life would not be worth living. Why not throw me away? After all, my life would be worthless since my body would be incapable of moving just like everyone else's. What good could come of a life unable to measure up to society's standards? But such standards of measurement never take into account the reality of love. Those who wanted to throw me away failed to realize that in my broken body lives a human being with a soul who is able to love, think, and be happy. For Socrates, the great philosopher of ancient Greece, only an examined life is worth living. And, yes, even according to this high standard, my life is worth living, because now I am a philosopher, a theologian, and a writer. I am living proof that no one can predict another's future. Often predictions fail because all the factors that form and influence a life are unknown. I've rivaled the predictions of many since being that young child. I've run and swam more miles than most, and earned several degrees: one in physical education and another in theology.

The doctor's determination that my life would be worthless comes as no surprise. Society values what is beautiful, strong, and graceful, and determines how these criteria are defined. We honor athletes who run the fastest and jump the farthest. We line up all the beauty queens to rate the most attractive. When we ask a pregnant woman or an expectant father, "What do you want, a boy or a girl?" the usual response is, "I don't care, as long as it's healthy." What if the baby isn't healthy? It is not wrong to desire a healthy baby; disability and illness are undesirable. The point is that most people don't fully consider the expectations they set up for their lives and families. Families often discover after having a child with a disability that they love the child no matter what.

So what would guide my parents to accept my brokenness and decide to keep me when many others listen to misguided advice? I believe that my parents learned something significant from their early lives. Not only did my father have the example of my uncle, but he also suffered much in his childhood. His father, a well-respected cobbler in Wakefield, a small town a few miles north of Boston, died of a heart attack at the age of fifty, leaving my grandmother a widow with seven children. My father, the youngest of them, was just six years old. Growing up in this difficult situation, my father learned an important lesson about what to do with brokenness. The answer is not to run away or to pretend that it does not exist. Rather, brokenness is to be faced head on. Wouldn't it have been better if his father had lived? Of course it would have, but my father and his family moved on in spite of the tragedy. So when it came time to make a decision about me, it really was no decision at all. My father knew what to do; he had to accept the brokenness and face it head on.

My mother suffered a similar fate in her childhood. Her father was forty-two years old when World War II broke out. He was too old to join the service, so he joined the Merchant Marines. As a mechanic who worked in the engine room, he was likely killed instantly when a torpedo hit his ship. My grandmother was notified of my grandfather's death on her oldest daughter's sixteenth birthday. My mother was just six years old when my grandmother found herself with eight little mouths to feed. In order to give her children a decent childhood, my grandmother relied on relatives, prayed, and worked. One day after she had prayed in desperation over how she would feed her children, she opened her living room window and found four twenty-dollar bills in her bushes. No one knows how they got there. The truth is, she was so desperate that she didn't care. All that mattered was that she now had enough money to feed her children for several weeks. My mother learned from my grandmother what to do in the face of suffering and brokenness. One uses whatever resources one has.

In Jewish folklore, before a person is born he or she looks down on earth and chooses his or her life circumstances. The soul decides the body and family of origin it wants. The soul sees the people who will give it the best opportunity to be the person it is meant to be, and it chooses these people for its family. It also chooses its body.[3] If I had such a choice, I am glad I made it the way I did, because my parents were exactly what I needed to have a chance at a full life. They knew how to turn and face my disability, because their earlier experiences had shown them how to deal with brokenness—not to be afraid or ashamed, but to face it head-on, knowing that eventually everything would be okay.

My parents knew that tragic events can be transformed. They would wait for this promise to show itself in my life as truly as they had seen it work in their own. My parents could have closed off my opportunities by complying with the doctor's suggestion to institutionalize me. Instead they decided with hope and faith that there was more to my life than the tragic event of my birth. They decided to keep possibilities for transformation alive. Their decision would mean hundreds of medical appointments, three surgeries, crutches, leg braces, and a host of other inconveniences and expenses. But the effort would pale in light of what they would receive in return. If my parents had institutionalized me, people could have come up to them and said, "It is truly a shame about your child." Instead, everyone met me as a bright-eyed, smiling child with a zest for life.

When tragic events occur, for whatever reason, we find ourselves lost in incomprehensible darkness, searching for adequate answers to changes thrust upon us without our consent or control. My parents were plunged into this darkness when cerebral palsy entered our lives forever. Filled with questions, my mother began to search for answers.

---

3. David A. Cooper, *Kabbalah Meditation: Judaism's Ancient System for Mystical Exploration through Meditation & Contemplation*, compact disc (Denver: Sounds True, 2004).

THE SEARCH FOR ANSWERS

In 1966 when I was first diagnosed, my mother went to the local library to find information on cerebral palsy. She found a thin pamphlet that said that only a small percentage of people with cerebral palsy are also mentally retarded. She was relieved to know that I probably would not have to struggle with cognitive as well as physical difficulties, although I know now that even if I had been developmentally delayed, everyone in my family would have loved me just the same.

Returning from the library, my mother must have pondered what she had to do. As only a parent can resolve, she must have made a silent commitment to give me the best life possible. I can imagine her pulling into our driveway and moving quietly and steadily toward our house, considering with each step the journey she was about to undertake. As she reached the front door, one of her other children probably ran out to greet her. As she picked up the child to play for a moment, she must have thought, "But how?"

I know her answer, because I lived it. My mother's answer was, "I will do this any way I know how, and with everything I have; and I will not let any one of my other children suffer as a result of this commitment." Indeed, my siblings never suffered or complained. God bless my mother and the dedication she carried for me. Sure, times would get tough between my mother and me in later years. Children and their mothers often disagree, but my mother's commitment was unmistakably to help me make the most of my life for the good of our entire family.

In keeping with this commitment, my mother began setting me outside to play in the yard while she did her housework. I was only four years old, but she figured I would have to learn to fend for myself in this dog-eat-dog world, so the lessons might as well start early. The trouble was that my mother never got much housework done when she did this. She spent more time peeking through her blinds to check on me than she spent vacuuming her carpet. One day I staggered around the yard, falling about every three steps, repeating, "Here, kitty, kitty." It was such a pretty black kitty with a lovely white stripe down its back. My mother was there in a flash. "That's not a kitty," she said as she came up behind me, swooped me up in her arms, and scurried back into the house. On that day, my mother was thankful for my tortoise-like speed, because at the rate I was going, I would never have caught up with that baby skunk.

When I was three years old, I got my first set of crutches and leg braces. One day my mother received a pink order slip from the doctor, and we went to a dungeon-like basement workshop. I remember its being incredibly dark except for a light that shone from an old desk lamp. Crumpled old pink slips covered the desk, which was pushed up against a high workbench. Crutches and parts of old braces hung on the walls, and shoes were scattered everywhere. I remember the place being scary, but the "brace man" was kind and gentle, and I felt more comfortable after he greeted us. My mother handed him the slip, along with an extra pair of my shoes.

Night after night, my mother must have tossed and turned, thinking, "Will tomorrow be the day those braces will be ready and my daughter will walk without her crutches?" When the day finally came, she must have thought, "Today my daughter will take those first beautiful and wonderful steps." She must have imagined the wonder of my first few steps as if I were a one-year-old, even though I was nearly four.

As my mother recounts the story, she rushed home and immediately put the braces on me. Designed to get my feet to point outward instead of inward, they had metal rods on each side of my shoes that reached to just below my knees and attached to a leather cuff that wrapped around my calf. She stood me with my back to the refrigerator so I could walk toward her out into the open kitchen. With my mother and my new braces supporting me, I stood without my crutches. She let go and backed away, so I could take my first magical steps. I teetered for a moment—and fell over.

We laughed, as we always did when I fell, and although I don't remember it, I'll bet my mother cried. She had expected these new braces to make me normal. The braces would indeed make my life better, but not normal.

Now, as I tell this story, I can feel my mother's heartbreak. She longed for me to have a life filled with movement, fun, and, yes, normality. She was determined to give me whatever I needed to advance myself in life. Her commitment was the driving force that made my excursions in both the front yard and the backyard possible. Fortunately she received some truly life-saving advice from my neurologist. Dr. Barrenberg, director of the neurology department at Harvard Medical School, told her to treat me like all her other children. My mother took this advice to an extreme. She used every opportunity to say to me, "You are no different from the others."

One day we came out of a discount store with a green jump rope in my hand and flip-flop sandals on my feet. Jumping rope and wearing flip-flop sandals were both out of the question. My mother put those flip-flop sandals, with only one prong between the big toe and the second toe, back on my feet more times than I can count. My toes could not grip the prong so off the sandals would go, and my mother, God bless her, would just put them back on me. As for jumping rope, I think I managed at best three consecutive jumps, and that was a great accomplishment.

Even though jumping rope and wearing flip-flops were impossible for me, the rope and the sandals were a testimony to what my mother was trying to tell me. By her actions, she was communicating, "You can do anything and everything you put your mind to." I know to some this may seem unbelievable, but my mother often demanded the impossible from me, and sometimes she got it. I echoed this sentiment to the psychologist who evaluated my IQ when I was four years old. During the examination, as my medical records from Children's Hospital attest, I kept saying to the psychologist, "Watch, I can do everything!" My parents must have been proud and relieved when the report came back saying, "Superior intelligence, much higher than average." My intellect would not be the problem; my struggle would be to move.

The parameters of my struggle were becoming clearer. I would not be healed instantly with my new braces. Now it was time to pursue the best and most meaningful life possible, and this would mean surgery. The doctors wanted to surgically stretch my tendons in an attempt to undo some effects of the spasticity brought on by the cerebral palsy.

Much to my dismay, the call to go under the knife came sooner rather than later. As a child of four, I was so scared, that I ran a fever on the day I was scheduled to be admitted to the hospital. I remember leaving the house with my siblings all lined up waving goodbye, only for my parents and me to pull into the driveway a few hours later without my having had surgery. I felt a sense of triumph when surgery was canceled that day, but I did not know that my hope never to have surgery would soon be dashed. My siblings and I had a few more days to play and have fun together, and then I was again hauled off to the hospital against my will.

A CRY FOR COMFORT

I wait, terrified, thinking about the surgery in the morning. What will happen to me? The rails of my hospital bed hem me in where I don't want to be. Every once in a while, I think, "If I could just climb out, I would be able to free myself." But there is no way out. I am trapped with nowhere to go, and tomorrow the doctors will cut me open. I know Curious George ate the puzzle piece and the doctors got it out of his stomach, but for right now, I am scared. It doesn't matter that Curious George was okay. I want to be okay right now, and I am not. I want to leave, but my mother is nowhere to be found.

The room is lined with rows of hospital beds, and the lights are dimmed so all the little children can sleep. But who can find rest? How can I? My mind is filled with terror. There is no comfort to absorb the uncertainty of tomorrow's surgery. Tears begin to stream down my face. A deep sense of aloneness seizes my soul. My mind says, "There is no one here—no comfort, no touch, and no mother."

Tears begin to well up inside me as I whisper these words, "Mommy, Mommy, Ma, Ma." I squeeze the life out of my little blankie, pulling it tighter and closer toward me. Louder and louder my cries become as the other children toss in their beds. My body violently trembles. As my cries become more forceful, my mind chimes in, "Is she coming? Is she here yet?" Then another thought crosses my mind: maybe if I am quiet she will come and comfort me. With a strength not quite my own comes a resolve to be quiet. This calms my shaking body. "Shhhh, shhhh. Quiet. Maybe this will help. Just be calm for a few minutes," I say to myself. Quietly, I begin to wait. No mother, no mother, there is no mother. She is not here. No one is here. I am all alone! The tide of tears rushes back.

Aloneness and fear grip my soul as if to snicker, "Now I've got you and you can't get away."

"No, no. No mother, no mother to rescue me," I say to myself. "No mother; she is not coming," my heart echoes as I peer through the wide doorway into the dimly lit hallway. I see only emptiness and a small spot of reflected light on the shiny white-tile floor. Aloneness brings anger as tears again trickle and fall, streaming down to stain my pillow. Violent outbursts of rage accompany my tears as if to say, "Hear my cry, hear it now! I will make it so loud, you will not be able to ignore it!" Again I clutch my blankie as tightly as I can, as if to squeeze out all the reassurance it can offer. I wish my blankie could tell me, "It's going to be okay."

But even my trusty blankie leaves me with no reassurance. My mind rages helplessly. "Take me home—I don't want to be here! What will happen to me tomorrow? This is not fair! Get me out of here! Please let me go!"

Nothing works, and my crying continues. Suddenly I see movement in the hall. "Look, here comes a nurse! Maybe she can help," my mind says, and my heart feels a glimmer of hope. The nurse walks to my bedside and glances down at my poor, small, broken, half-naked body shaking from all the tears and anger. "Now, you be quiet. Hush," she says. "Don't make me come in here again!" She turns from me and walks like a general past the shiny spot on the floor, disappearing from my view.

Why didn't an army of angels swoop down from heaven to comfort me? Why didn't the nurse who came to check on me provide me with soft words of comfort? Where were the hands of God when a contorted little body cried out for love and found none? What does it mean that God dwells in the darkness, in our deepest wounds? Why didn't God address my neediness? Couldn't divine wisdom and infinite love have provided me with what I needed on the spot and in an instant?

After many years, God would begin to provide me with answers to the pain I experienced that night. Even in the depths of our darkness when we cannot know God, we unknowingly receive comfort.

Sometimes life feels like a barren wasteland where we long for love, but find none. Why is love missing? As I searched for answers, I began to understand how God meets us in our pain. The Scriptures tell us that God is love. I believe I experienced God in the darkness as I waited for my mother to arrive, even though I was not conscious of it at the time. In some mysterious way, love was with me even though it remained incomprehensible to me.

It is as if the darkness speaks. "Trust the darkness! Trust your soul!" it says.

We ask God, "Where is the intimacy? Where is the love?"

"Here I am. I am hiding in the darkness," God says.

As we dare to believe that God is in the darkness, love begins to take hold. As I reflected on the loss of that night years later, I felt a touch of love deep inside, even in my darkest, most private pain. "No, no, this can't be true. I am in too much pain," I said to myself. My pain and aloneness continued, and my need for intimacy still raged strong, but something else was with it. When we dare to believe that God dwells in the darkness, tiny moments of love touch us and bring us comfort. These moments express the sacred paradox that light lives in darkness, and that darkness never has the power to overcome it completely.

When we trust that God dwells in the darkness, love appears. Where else would God choose to dwell? God always communicates love, so of course God would want to proclaim love in our deepest wounds. God does this even though we are unable to recognize God's light shining through the darkness. When we experience God in the darkness, we find God dwelling in our pain. God communicates love even though the love remains hidden and incomprehensible to us. In the darkness God addresses our pain, albeit indirectly. We want God to swoop down from heaven with miraculous power to take our suffering away, but that does not happen. Instead, we must live with our brokenness, believing that God is with us in our pain. The happy and hopeful news is that God never stops giving. God always provides a way for us to know divine love.

In the midst of pain we must remember God. It is only by remembering and knowing God that we gain power to move beyond the tragedy invading our lives. During our episodes of pain, God illuminates us from within, revealing new truths and new mysteries. We enter into these mysteries when we meditate on God in light of the tragic event and the resulting experience of suffering and brokenness.

Tragedy sneaks up on us like a thief in the night, stealing our preconceived notions about what our lives ought to be and leaving us struggling to find answers as we examine the shattered pieces of our lives. Here in the ruins, we must pick up the fragments of our broken world to begin anew.

Tragedy makes us angry and forces us to question God. To end the anger that we carry toward our tragic situation and God the only thing I know to do is to turn humbly toward God and ask, "Lord God, how can we live now?"

Our new reality of brokenness and suffering will at first appear to be only a disastrous fate. In time, however, something more of life's unfolding plan will reveal itself. Out of the depths of tragedy, new life will begin. We will hear the whisper of a mysterious and secret blessing hiding in the scattered ruins of our lives.

The only way I know to continue our lives in spite of our tragedy is to remind ourselves that God is with us, and that God gives us new lives with new possibilities.

TWO

Exploring the Possibilities

THROUGHOUT MY CHILDHOOD, THE memory of the night before my surgery made me feel abandoned. Why God does not intervene to prevent horrific and tragic events remains a mystery. Yes, natural laws govern the universe, and God does not usually override these laws, but the question, why? constantly haunts us as we try to deal with tragedy in our lives. When we are in pain, we hope for instant healing. Isn't that what God is supposed to do? And so we cry out, "Heal me now, God!"

Life rarely works that way, although miracles have been known to happen. It is true, I must admit, that at times I want a magical God. I want a God who will give me exactly what I want, the way I want it. I want everything to be just the way I would like it to be. "Voilà! Alakazam!" I would say, and the world would conform to my every wish.

But if we cannot prevent tragedy and adversity, we most of the time have the power to choose our responses and plan our actions. The greatest choice we can make when we are struck down is to decide to rise again and not to let tragedy have the final word. To do this, we must be willing to act in small ways to change our lives in spite of what looks so bleak all around us. It is here, in the midst of so much pain, that we must find the strength to turn to God, believing that God is with us in our trial.

When tragedy strikes, our beliefs about God often get knocked out of whack. We begin to question God: "God, why didn't you . . .?" I feel your rage because I have had it, too: It says, "If God is with me, then why am I forced to live this way?" When our prayers for healing remain unanswered, it is difficult to understand. Doesn't God care? Is God unable to intervene? Why was this tragedy thrust upon me? What gives death and tragedy the right to disturb life? Where is God? Over and over again, these questions roll around in our minds, disturbing us and leaving us with ever more doubt. This doubt snatches from us our belief that God loves and cares for us.

Though we cannot know the reason for our loss, we can hold to this truth: life is asking us to move on and live in the midst of our tragic circumstances. We need to lay aside life as it should have been and accept, as best we can, reality as it is. It's not that we accept our lives completely once and for all and never have to revisit the issue again. Rather, as we crack the door of acceptance to our new life, we give God an opportunity to be with us through our painful hardships.

AFTER THE FIRST SURGERY

After my first surgery, designed to allow me to separate my legs, I returned home in a cast that reached to my waist. When my father and mother brought me into the house, they had to tilt me sideways because the cast separating my legs was wider than the doorway. They carried me upstairs to the bedroom as if I were a piece of furniture, and both blew a sigh of relief when they reached my little bed. Pillows surrounded me in my crib, which would be my new home for nearly six months.

The cast separated into two halves. In the beginning, both halves needed to stay on, and I really couldn't move. (There were holes in the cast so I could go to the bathroom.) When it was time, my mother would take the top half off and stretch my legs. She often reminded me that when I was a baby, it was very difficult to pry my spastic legs apart so that she could change my diaper.

In the crib alone, I experienced much silence. In the silence, I learned to listen. Hearing the commotion of my siblings at play often inspired my imagination to create the scenes of their play in my mind. My imagination showed me all the ways I wished to move but could not.

In the silence I also learned to find God through the early stirrings of my soul. Although I had no words for it at the time, I would feel God's love touching me in the silence. My experience of love would come through encountering God and also through the actions of others. My longing for love on the night before my surgery made me keenly aware of and able to recognize even the slightest trace of affection moving in my direction. I could always, with joy, detect footsteps as they made their way up the stairs toward the bedroom. Being able to listen for God and others allowed me to unearth the endless possibilities that life gives in spite of painful losses.

Many visitors came to see me in those first few days and scrawled their names across my cast. My brother Bernie, the rebel teenager, signed the bum part. After a few days, the visitors thinned out. Back then, my days were spent with my record player or in the quiet. One special visitor always filled my heart with joy. He would come and stand by my crib and play the staring game. Nose against nose, each player was to stare into the other person's eyes and not blink. If you blinked before the other person did, you lost. Of course, as I stared into my Uncle Paul's hazel eyes, I would always blink before he did. We would laugh. Sometimes he would bring me something special like a stuffed animal, but other times, he would just bring himself. Either way, I felt special and loved because my Uncle Paul visited me. This happy experience with him stood in stark contrast to my feeling abandoned in my hospital bed.

Often, simple acts of love make a great deal of difference. This is my Uncle Paul's talent. He fixes cars for a living and does a great job of it. Much more important than the wrench in his hand or the grease under his fingernails is the warmth in his soul that motivates him to do little things with great care. We get caught up in all kinds of things that are unimportant; we say that we are too busy. My uncle knew that the little postwork detail—namely, his niece—was important. He could have been "too busy" to come and see me after working hard all day. But without his visits, I would have been untouched by his love, and that love wouldn't have helped me get past the abandonment I had felt so deeply just days earlier. My uncle helped me find new possibilities of love.

It takes many people to initiate healing. It still pleases me immensely that my uncle helped healing possibilities come to life within me. No one could have imagined how great the possibilities would be.

A short twelve years later, Uncle Paul greeted me joyfully as I ran past his garage during a three-and-a half mile run. How happy and proud he must have been to contrast the two scenes—the one of me being unable to move in a cast, and the other of me nearly whizzing by his shop, hardly wanting to stop. I stared into my uncle's eyes as he held his wrench in his hand, ready to get back to work. His eyes shut before mine did, but I think he let me win that time. That dose of love from my uncle's heart made the mile run home feel like I was floating on air. I see the two scenes in my mind and my disabled legs become like a pair of wings. No one would have predicted that I'd be running.

The road to my long-distance runs was paved with many difficult trials. My mother and I logged many long hours of physical therapy as we fought against a tide of doubters who preferred emphasizing my diminished capacity, rather than helping unearth my beautiful potential. We discovered early that, although tragedy had struck, life would always hold some new possibility for transformation. Years later, these possibilities would become clear as I learned to seek the inexhaustible love of God even in my pain.

We will begin to seek God's love in our pain when we can acknowledge that suffering is part of life. Although we cannot know why we have been unjustly singled out, we can still accept that God has a sacred purpose for our lives, as God does for every one. We can get to this point of accepting our situation only by adopting an attitude of nonviolence toward our own being and toward our feelings of self-contempt. With a soft loving hand, we must reach within ourselves to soothe our inner wounds. We do this by listening to ourselves—our thoughts, feelings, and complaints—not reminiscing over what is lost, but looking forward to what remains in spite of the loss. Once we can do this, we are close enough to acceptance of our situation to hear the still, small whisper of God. The faint murmuring that we hear brings forth our knowledge of God's redemptive purpose in this world and the next. Attuned to God's quiet voice, although we suffer innocently, we are able to turn toward God in our pain to find a wellspring of consolation.

As I learned to listen to God speaking through silence and to my own experiences of brokenness, I would discover the essence of hope. Hope believes in future possibilities. Josef Pieper, a German philosopher, describes hope as the anticipation of fulfillment.[1] To have hope is to be like a pilgrim: to be as one on his or her way, willing to accept the "not yet" character of life. The pilgrim walks forward, willing to embrace that the future is unknown and thus holds out the possibility for new life. The pilgrim believes that as long as there is breath, there is opportunity for transformation. As long as life lasts, life can be renewed. It takes a soul who courageously seeks what is best to bring this kind of hope to life—one who, in spite of tragic circumstances, is willing to step out in anticipation that something better and more remarkable exists, even when such a dream seems unreal and impossible.

1. Josef Pieper, *On Hope* (San Francisco: Ignatius, 1986) 65.

LISTENING FOR GOD

This is the key: once we understand how God relates to our tragedy, then we are able to experience God even though we suffer. First we must keep in mind that suffering is part of the fabric of our universe, and we must embrace the truth that, though we can influence our lives, we are not in complete control of all events that happen to us. When we think we control our destinies, we consider ourselves more highly than we ought, for humankind has always been inescapably finite. Our limits are clear at the moment of the fateful diagnosis or the unfortunate accident.

Knowing that suffering is part of the landscape of our existence allows us to accept our situation. It makes us willing to work within the confines of our suffering, and this ultimately leads to a connection with God and the transformation we seek. When we have prayed for healing and an answer does not come, it is likely that God is calling us to take a journey to find inner healing. This inner healing is not like the miracles of Jesus, which were accompanied by outward signs and instant cures. Inner healing comes to us when we know the healing touch of God *in spite of* the persistence of our ailments.

How do we find this healing from within? How do we know the living love of God even though pain disturbs us? Healing is a journey, one that we do not take once and for all. Rather, we continually travel through the things that hurt us in the hope that our pain will be relieved. The journey begins within the heart. As the heart seeks to be healed, a deep longing for love wells up inside it. The pilgrimage continues with a commitment to the healing process. Each pilgrim must be completely mindful of God on his or her way. Each careful step is taken in devotion to God.

And then one day our pain, suffering, and anguish are surpassed. A joyful refrain fills the heart, and it says, "How great is God!" We reach the destination when we can say, "This pain that I carry, although it is still pain, disturbs me no longer." Our suffering is transformed: we still experience and know our pain, but we find our way beyond its unbearable aspects so that it conveys a different message.

Times of healing, however, are momentary treasures. For once inner healing is found in one area of brokenness, another aspect of pain quickly emerges. The pilgrim must remain committed; soon he or she will depart on a new journey through some other pain.

Pilgrimage need not be lonely. I've made many friends along the way who remind me that God's love is our surest and most enduring reality. Not that I knew of them during the early days of my pain. Rather, the truth about which they wrote was alive and with me throughout my journey. Thus I have repeatedly turned to them, as to good friends, for comfort and solace. As I am a pilgrim on my own healing journey, these authors are the companions of my heart. Their voices speak to me, and their words remind me of God's love as I seek a way to inner healing amid suffering, pain, and brokenness.

I first met Carlo Carretto (1910–1988) through his most popular book, *Letters from the Desert*. In clear, crisp, poetic language he expresses how he heard God's voice. In turn, he teaches us how to listen and hear too. Carretto shared his life with the poorest of the poor who live in the Sahara Desert, forgotten by the modern world. At the age of forty-four, he heard God's call: "Leave everything; come with me into the desert. I don't want your action any longer. I want your love."[2] Having earned a doctoral degree in philosophy from the University of Turin, Carretto left Italy in obedience to the voice. He went to the desert to join the Little Brothers of Jesus, a religious order founded by Charles de Foucauld. Besides a strict commitment to serve the poor as one of them, the Little Brothers of Jesus seek to model their lives in very concrete ways after the life of Jesus.

Carretto's words penetrate the soul with such force that readers are challenged to think seriously about how far they might be willing to carry their own commitment to God. As I read his words, I began to say to myself, "Oh God, if this is what is required, and if this is how I am living, I am sorry, so sorry." How many of us would be willing to give up our modern lives to live in the Sahara Desert with the poorest of the poor, in order to model our lives radically after that of Jesus? We are all challenged every day, yet how many of us are willing to set aside our own personal agendas in order to accept our everyday trials?

Once his initial training in the Sahara Desert was over, Carretto dreamed of being part of the Alpine rescue teams that work on the Matterhorn. He hoped to move back to the western Alps, along the border between southwest Switzerland and northwest Italy, to fulfill his obligations as a Little Brother of Jesus closer to home. Carretto and a friend, who was also a male nurse, went hiking in the desert one day. Carretto

2. Carlo Carretto, *Letters from the Desert*, trans. Rose Mary Hancock (Maryknoll, NY: Orbis, 1976) xvii.

was not in good physical shape for hiking, so his friend said, "I'll give you some shots. You'll see; they'll keep you going." Carretto agreed, and in less than twenty-four hours, his leg was useless. The nurse had used the wrong vial and injected Carretto's thigh with a paralyzing poison.

Carretto tried to keep cheerful even though the accident would leave his leg paralyzed for life. He writes in *Why O Lord*, "It was stupid, but I would not say the nurse had been at fault except in the sense that he was impulsive and careless. I didn't complain then, and I tried to keep cheerful if only to help the nurse whose fault it was not to go out of his mind."[3] And because of that terrible mistake, he bid farewell to any hope of ever climbing the Matterhorn.

"Suddenly I felt cheated. How could I be betrayed in this way? I'd come to Africa to become a Little Brother. I'd wanted to devote myself to the people dying in the snowstorms. I wanted to save them. Had I been wrong about that? . . . How could the God I wanted to serve not reach out his hand when I needed him? Why didn't he step in and stop such a simple, stupid mistake? Why didn't he help me? . . . Here I come to serve him, and all he seems to do is mock me and turn me into a cripple."[4]

Carretto abandoned his life as a social activist for a life completely dedicated to prayer and communion with God, and God allowed tragedy to strike. It is difficult to comprehend, but Carretto, with his wisdom and love for God, points the way to acceptance and healing transformation. In spite of feeling cheated, he shows us that the paralysis held for him an important lesson. He writes, "I have experienced in my flesh what Augustine says: 'God permits evil, so as to transform it into a greater good.'"[5]

After thirty years, Carretto describes the paralysis as a misfortune that God transformed into a grace:

"Thirty years have passed since then—thirty years after my dream went wrong . . . It was bad luck, yes. It was a misfortune. But God turned it into a grace. I had a useless leg. I could not climb. So I got a jeep and became a meteorologist. Through no wish of my own I was where I belonged: in the desert."[6]

---

3. Carlo Carretto, *Why O Lord? The Inner Meaning of Suffering*, trans. Robert R. Barr (Maryknoll, NY: Orbis, 1986) 4.

4. Ibid., 4–5.

5. Ibid., 7.

6. Ibid., 6.

When he says he became a meteorologist, Carretto does not mean that he took to delivering tomorrow's weather on the evening news. Carretto is talking about what he calls the friendly night. The night is friendly in the desert because stars tell us how to find our way. Carretto would use stars as a guidance system to find his way so he could come to the aid of his brothers living among the native tribes in various areas of the desert. He would also use his meteorological skills to predict the weather so he would be better able to provide supplies for his brothers as they fulfilled their calling to live out their lives as Christ's servants among the poorest of the poor.

Carretto's accident kept him in the desert with his jeep, his eyes turned to the sky. It enabled him to become a shepherd to his brothers. He learned from his wounds the beauty of sacrifice and how to serve his brothers. He in turn teaches us that our pain can bring to us knowledge of God. Through the power of God's grace, a tragic event was transformed into a healing journey. Now that Carretto was not going to be the mountain climber of his dreams, he began to hear the desert inviting him into silence and prayer. Having found God in the midst of his suffering, he realized, "You can be very happy with a crippled leg. Very happy."[7]

What is most important in finding one's way to transformation? Carretto emphasizes an experience with God. That is exactly what I found after my first surgery. Through the murmurings of our household and the visitors who came to share love and hope with me, I had an experience with God that would lead me to transformation. Like Carretto, whose new life was thrust upon him as a result of a tragic event, I would find a new way of being and thinking because of what I lost at my birth. My new life would be a battle, not a picnic. My brokenness would mean not only the loss of physical ability but also, in some instances, the diminishment of love.

I first realized this loss of love on the night of my first surgery, when my mother wasn't with me though I needed her so desperately. Over and over again I wondered why such basic comfort was denied me. If God wasn't going to give me a normal body, at least God could have provided me with the comfort and love necessary to endure it. As Carretto and I both know, history cannot be undone. When tragedy strikes, it leaves its mark forever. But its consequences need not remain unchanged. God would

7. Ibid., 7.

reveal to me the truth of which Carretto speaks: that trials are infused with opportunities for God's grace and love. Although I did not know it at the time, my early loss of comfort would become the foundation of my spiritual life. My insatiable longing for love would be directed toward the Holy One of Israel, the Lord our God. My almost constant desire would become my great teacher, pointing me toward God with each new manifestation of my neediness. And through the silence, I would come to know perhaps the most important truth: God would never leave me to endure my pain alone. God would join me on a pilgrimage, a healing journey that would transform my suffering.

Healing comes when we are ever mindful of the possibilities and goodness that surround us every day, no matter what our circumstances. We must keep in mind the truth that we are not in complete control of our lives. Tragedy can strike through no fault of our own. Whether we like it or not, suffering, pain, and struggles are part of the fabric of our everyday lives. Whatever our circumstances, we are given the power to choose: we can try to curtail the effects of our suffering, or we can succumb to the pain and let it have the final word. Not surrendering to the pain would be very important to me, because my cerebral palsy would require many long hours of physical therapy.

PHYSICAL THERAPY

I remember my mother bringing me to the basement of Children's Hospital for my physical-therapy appointments. Today my siblings are with me. They are all sitting in little chairs lined up around the perimeter of the therapy room.

These are not the days of casual sneakers and blue jeans. My siblings are wearing their Sunday best on a weekday—a must for my mother back in 1968. My brothers, seven-year-old Joe and five-year-old Paul, are sporting bright red wool blazers with a black and gold coat of arms sewn on the breast pocket. Their shiny black shoes restlessly tap the floor as they wait for the whole ordeal to be over. "How long will this punishment of sitting still in our Sunday clothes have to continue?" they must wonder as they work hard to stay in their chairs and quietly behave. My sisters, eight-year-old Mariann and six-year-old Sue, are wearing colorful dresses and have ribbons in their hair. Their white shoes dangle and swing aimlessly.

After sneaking a glimpse at them, I realize it is time to get on with my work. I focus my attention back on Miss Lane, my physical therapist. With her kitty eyeglasses whose corners point straight up into the air, she looks mean and scary. My mother watches Miss Lane intently, no doubt hoping her four other children will behave for the remainder of my physical-therapy session. An emergency with the babysitter must have arisen. Instead of canceling my appointment, my mother, God bless her soul, brought us all.

Miss Lane begins to instruct my mother as I was lying down on the physical-therapy table, "You raise her leg up and put it on your shoulder. Once the leg is there, have her press down. Diana, press down." I press my leg into her shoulder. "Okay, stop once she stops. Push your shoulder into her leg to raise it up even higher. You see, this stretches the hamstring muscles in the back of the leg. Now you take her leg and try."

Miss Lane guides my mother through her first attempts at the exercise. The two of them put me through my paces, getting me to do this exercise and then another. As fatigue sets in, I keep plugging along, silent and uncomplaining. My siblings, whatever they are doing, are far from me as I concentrate with all my might on performing the exercises with perfection. As I am being commanded to move this way and that, I wonder what new impossible moves Miss Lane and my mother will invent. Each new exercise makes me want to say, "You want me to do *what*?" Take my right leg and put it behind my earlobe—yeah, right. The routine exercises are bad enough: "Kick your leg out straight while I try to push down on it. Now, ready, set, go!"

By this time, my brothers are getting restless. When all my prone exercises are finished and I move to the edge of the examining table, they spring from their seats as if finally released from punishment. They begin to explore the gym-like atmosphere with its pulleys, parallel bars, mirrors, mats, and other exercise equipment. Soon they are walking carefully between the parallel bars. Heel and then toe. After they take their initial steps, they watch themselves in the mirror. They spin effortlessly and confidently back and forth between the bars as if to say, "See, I've got this walking thing down pat."

As long as her sons do not disturb anything, my mother lets them play. She knows that the few moments of quiet she has stolen are far more than she can expect. Now we enter the middle of the room in the midst of my brothers' game, and they will have to turn the parallel bars over to me so I can walk without my crutches. The physical therapist carefully adjusts the bars on either side of me to fit my small frame. She instructs me to use a heel-toe motion. I etch into my mind my brother Joe's steps as he had effortlessly moved between the bars just moments before. His ease at walking is a far cry from my own clumsy steps, but with my mother and my physical therapist watching, I know I have to try. *Can't* is a four-letter word in my young vocabulary, so, marching off, I look into the mirror for a miracle.

My feet scrape the wooden boards between the bars as I make my way back and forth. With each pass, Miss Lane and my mother issue a new set of instructions. Each command makes me try harder. Though I cannot match my brother's perfect steps, I fix them in my mind to use as a model at a later date. As I walk, Miss Lane scribbles down a new set of exercises, complete with instructional stick figures. My mother and I will work on these at home. Soon my mother takes the sheet, gathers her entourage of finely dressed little ones, and returns home to continue her duties as a top-notch domestic engineer.

After my physical-therapy sessions, my mother would lay me on the kitchen table to begin my exercises again, rehearsing each sequence as if she were getting ready for the lead part in a play.

"Okay, raise up, press down, and I'll stretch." Up, down, and all around we would go. While my mother was pushing and prodding me to undo my disability, I often wished she could have recognized my painful struggle. Could she have shown me a softer, gentler, kinder self that would also have pushed me forward? Her hands touched me as she held my legs in the air, but they never expressed the depth of feeling I needed or wanted. They never reached through to my pain, through to the struggle of trying, always trying to be better and to do more. My mother did not see that I was getting lost in the conquest of "being able to" as I strove to make new things happen. Never was I free from the constant drive to be much more than I was; my life never offered me freedom to let go and simply be a child. Even my world of play was invaded by the challenge of walking to the sandbox or making my way to the swings. My mother's hands manipulated me for my benefit, but she knew nothing of my deep inner pain.

The pain followed me everywhere, moment by moment, day by day, challenging me to cope with the changes that I had been given without my consent. This pain, my inner pain, would gnaw at me, taunting me and ridiculing me whenever it got a chance: "I am your pain, and you can't do anything about me." I longed for my mother to recognize how deeply I wanted to be like my siblings. Ah, to run and play just like them! More than anything, I needed her to touch the pain of realizing that my walking would never be like that of everyone else. I would have liked to hear, "You're stiff today; maybe I am pushing too hard. Do your legs hurt? Are you in pain?" At least that would have reached through to the part of me that was in physical pain. Even more amazing would have been for her to recognize and touch my inner pain by saying something like, "Was it hard for you today at physical therapy to see your siblings walk?" The simple acknowledgement of my feelings would have gone a long way toward helping to heal my inner pain.

Living without any recognition of my painful situation forced me to work hard to please my mother. Maybe if I worked hard enough, my disability and brokenness would go away and she would be satisfied. My father also was a great fan of hard work. He wanted me, and all his children, always to do our best. Had any one of us brought home a report card with straight *D*s, but with all *A*s for effort, he would have praised us for trying hard. So, wanting to please both my parents as much as I wanted to curtail the effects of my disability, I always gave my exercises my best effort.

In defense of my mother, I don't think she intentionally neglected my feelings. She was on a mission from God to give me life through helping me develop my ability to move, and she did not fail. She taught me with great care, and in later years the results of her care would leave doctors and physical therapists in awe. Every day I live off the benefits of her efforts by moving anywhere I want to go. I've scaled mountains and swum my way through some rivers and streams. I've run and walked far more miles than my siblings—more than anyone ever would have dreamed—because my mother worked on me on the kitchen table, day after day, tirelessly, no doubt saying to herself and believing, "I will help this situation. I will take action to make it change." I've seen many children whose mothers did not make the same effort, and they for sure don't share the same freedom of movement that I enjoy.

So it is not surprising if in her tireless effort to "make it change," my mother sometimes failed to realize the depth of my personal struggle. Her inability to address my feelings and emotions fueled even further my longing for love. Fortunately, God would begin where my mother's ability to help me left off. My heart longed to make sense of my pain but didn't know how. Luckily, God showed me how.

God created in me the desire to look, to know, and to listen. Somehow, by perhaps the greatest miracle of my life, I could hear and respond to God. This does not mean that I heard God speak in a booming voice, or that I walked around with a glowing halo around my head. The voice I heard in those early days, and still hear today, is born of a deep listening and brings me to a spiritual place. As the challenges of my early life with a disability mounted up, I learned to hear God and to respond to the divine voice from the depths of my inner being.

Physically I progressed rapidly, doing things that no one ever dreamed I could do. The trouble was that, even though I overcame limitations every day, new limits were ever with me. And as I longed for comfort in the midst of these challenges, my mother's firm hand relentlessly pushed me ever harder. Constantly I would overcome something difficult only to find myself pressed up against a wall of another limitation. The boundary between what I could do and what I couldn't do felt like it would destroy my spirit until I would break through to the other side. And there I would find yet another boundary that could not easily be crossed.

It was always seemingly simple stuff: sit up straight, use your crutches, don't hyperextend your knees, raise your leg higher, and hold the stretch longer. On and on it went, every day. The limits that nagged at me, refusing to budge in the midst of the pressure, threatened to rob me of my connection with God. And this made me cry out, "Why me, God? Why me?"

My rage at God seemed endless even though I was always grateful for the miracles I had received. Sometimes all my efforts were futile, and my work did not give me the results I wanted. Frustrated, pressed up against an unyielding limit, I would find myself hating God. "Why can't I keep up with my brothers and sisters?" became my refrain.

And of course I hated myself for everything that I could not overcome. Yet despite my rage and a momentary loss of my connection with God, my journey continued, with its unremitting daily demands. In my young world, there simply was no avenue of escape. I could not give up. My hard efforts would have to continue in spite of the changing tides and storminess of my soul.

Even though my mother was intent on pushing me as hard as she could, some days she had just too much to do with her six other children. On those days she would send me into the den to do my exercises with

Maggie Lettvin, who did stretching exercises on our public television station, WGBH in Boston. I would follow along with Maggie, trying my best and then trying even harder to do the exercises just as Maggie did. God bless my mother, because she would have me believe that I could follow along. And indeed I could—to a point, and no further. This seemed to be the story of my life: always making it to a point, and no further. Whenever I wanted to stretch a little more to make my body more like that of the thin, agile woman I saw on the television screen, I careened out of control and crashed into my limits.

How pointless never to have perfection, never to have done it just right, never to have complete and total excellence, always to attain what we push for to a point, just so far, and no further; the dreaded limit, the dreaded body, the dreaded brokenness constantly holding us back, keeping us from our dreams! What is the real meaning of our limitations? Doesn't God want to teach us something more than self-hatred? Over and over again, God sends us back to our limits, where we can do things only up to a point and no further, to teach us the sacred lessons lying just below the depths of our imperfections that seem so unsightly to us.

ON THE EDGE

The newest little swimmers line up on the edge of the YMCA pool. The swimmers don't know status distinctions; soon, however, titles will become very important. The swimmers begin as mere "tadpoles," soon rise to "polliwogs," and then move up to "frog" and even "shark" status. Five years old, I am eager to become a shark. "Kick, make a splash!" the instructor says.

I sit at the end of the line just beyond the strong little boy and the cute redheaded girl. "Splash," my mind says. "Make a splash!" All the other children make white mountains of splash. My little legs move and move, yet from my effort no white water materializes. Only rippling ringlets and soft humps of unbroken water surround my small, disabled feet. "Try harder! Try harder!" my mind urges.

Meanwhile the instructor shouts more commands that echo in the pool area: "Faster, slower, a little splash, a big splash . . ."

The other children effortlessly follow along. Looking down the line from where I sit, I see with amazement the large white mountains of water diminishing and growing again as the instructions change. In a fury,

I push my legs as hard as I can. Nothing but smooth, soft water dunes encircle my small, disabled feet. As whitewater beads from the other children land all around me, my mind presses harder: "Make a splash, make a splash, just make the water break."

How in the world did I get on the edge? My mother put me there. Was she trying to kill my spirit? No doubt her objective was that I learn to swim, and a swimming class is the logical place to start. So in spite of my cerebral palsy and my little shriveled legs, she signed me up and dressed me in my swimsuit that day. Apprehension must have filled her as she removed my braces with care and put them in a locker so no one would disturb them. As she carried me to the pool, she may have thought, "The other mothers don't carry their children, and yet I carry mine!" What was going through her mind as she sat me on the edge of the pool? Perhaps she said to herself, "Though my daughter can barely walk without her crutches, now I am going to sit her here so she can learn to swim." Regardless of her doubts and apprehension, my mother sat me on the edge, next to the cute red-haired girl. I wonder: was she prepared to discuss me as the next Olympic hopeful? Could she sit proudly and watch my ripples? Did her stomach turn and cringe at the sight of my unbroken water?

The soft, unbroken dunes reveal something about beauty. The smooth channels are a unique creation given by God. God looks at our seemingly feeble creations and simply smiles. God never limits us without also giving us an opportunity to create beauty from our limitations. Once we are willing to accept our brokenness, we must take the opportunities that are presented to us. This means being willing to accept the consequences of our efforts, no matter how meager those efforts might seem. This is what it means to be on the edge: to take chances and interact with our unfortunate circumstances, regardless of the outcome. Being on the edge gives us the opportunity to transform our brokenness into a beautiful creation. Being on the edge lets us experience life as it really is, with all its potential harm and good. Many so-called failures are actually forms of courage, invisible to a culture that worships conformity. It takes courage to make ripples.

Think for a moment about how much greater the world would be if we could apprehend the beauty of our ripples as God does. The world would blossom with new and beautiful love. Horror and anguish over being different would be rendered meaningless. More of us would be free to experience life with joy and peace. If we, as a society, could comprehend the beauty of the ripples, we would not demand conformity to just one standard of excellence (that white mountain of splash). Instead we would look for the creative genius in our differences, and we would gain a new perspective on beauty.

We cannot discover this beauty in the midst of difference unless we are steadfast in the face of adversity, and we cannot be steadfast unless we believe that something more than tragedy lives in our differences. Tragic events are always subject to interpretation. Our lives need not be defined by tragedy. As we live with and begin to make sense of the tragedy, its meaning is subject to change. For example, when a woman goes blind, she experiences her blindness as tragic. But as time goes on, she learns that she can live without her sight, and the significance of her blindness changes. As she learns to endure tragic circumstances, she interprets her situation differently, and her life takes on a more positive character.

It is always better not to have received tragedy than to have received it, to see than not to see, to walk on two sturdy legs than to be lame. The tragic remains tragic. Even though this is true, disability and brokenness do not need to be complete tragedies, for both disability and brokenness can hold secret and hidden blessings. Our thoughts and attitudes toward the tragedy tell us how we will fare under its weight and pressure. Even when there seems to be no blessing, it is possible to believe that some measure of blessing remains to be revealed. I've known this to work even in the direst circumstances such as terminal illness.

A dear friend of mine, Frances Innes-Mitchell, shared my plight: she was born with cerebral palsy. Years later she was diagnosed with cancer. Despite her afflictions, she had strong faith and many friends. Slowly her capacities were taken from her—first her ability to drive and to live on her own, and then her power to move around. Finally she was completely bedridden. Even though she was dying, she loved God, clung to what was positive, and shared love with her many visitors. Frances transformed the bleak situation of her terminal illness and coming death into a real testimony of faith. During her final days she told her friends, "I go to sleep every night resting in the arms of my Lord Jesus." By looking for the blessings in even the bleakest of circumstances, she taught many how to live faithfully as earthly life slips away.

Looked at in a certain way, life on the pool's edge is a blessing. Sitting there, I ponder a different kind of reality, because I was not made just like everyone else. I have more to think about, more to experience, and ultimately more to apprehend from the heart of God. There is always more to a situation than meets the eye. When we look beyond our preconceived notions about brokenness, we discover a hidden blessing and goodness that are given to us by the love of God. It is not suffering itself, but rather the way we interpret it, that determines its consequences. When we interpret suffering in light of the love of God, it is transformed.

There is more to healing than outward appearances and physical realities. In fact the most enduring, pure, and beautiful healing always originates within, and it is this inner healing that transforms suffering. Inner healing removes the sting of loss so we can find the treasure and the beauty that are always hidden underneath our suffering. Inner healing is about discovering the goodness that cannot help but give itself every day throughout the universe. We recognize it most concretely in nature. In spite of wars and rumors of wars, every twenty-four hours the sun rises and sets, the birds sing, and the seasons move one day closer to changing. This goodness moving through nature comes to us in the rain as well as the sunshine. Even if we go through our lives unaware of it, new goodness is being born every day. Because of this goodness, we are able to receive the gift of inner healing and the hidden blessing found in brokenness.

To know and experience this hidden blessing, we must shift our focus from the surface of things to a deeper, more spiritual level. There is great danger in looking too much on the surface: when we do so, we fail to know the truth. Inundated with visual stimuli that block the true self from shining through, we are spiritually impoverished, unable to see or comprehend deeper truth. The only way to cure this spiritual impoverishment is to find new ways to look beyond the clutter. But we are so busy running around, trying to make it to the top, that we fail to see the reality that is right before us. Feeling, as well as thought, takes us beyond our superficial vision and enables us to see the spiritual realm penetrating the whole world.

It is easy to remain narrow minded when we pay attention only to the world of concrete facts. This type of thought keeps us from seeing the hidden blessing that lives in our suffering and brokenness. But when we embrace spiritual reality, we are forced into a place where brokenness is accepted, known, and understood. Reaching this place is not an end, but a beginning.

The acceptance of brokenness assures us that mysteriously hidden in tragedy are new opportunities for growth. This change in perception illuminates new mysteries. It gives us the courage to look beyond what can be seen only concretely and to see into the spiritual realm, where we find reason to go on. Looking at our brokenness and suffering with a spiritual eye unveils the possibility of miracles. We begin to hope that our pain and suffering may not have the final word.

But we cannot take a step forward and make the most of our circumstances unless we let go of what "should have been" and accept our situation as it is. Acceptance allows God to meet us in our suffering. I began my healing journey after my first surgery when I learned to listen for God in silence. Carlo Carretto and I share the conviction that God never leaves us alone in our pain. So we must thoughtfully listen for God. The intimacy with God that follows this listening shows us that life always holds out for us some new opportunities for transformation. These possibilities become known to us through God's inexhaustible love.

I found these opportunities in the everyday experiences of my childhood. Through the pool's edge with its unbroken water, I discovered spiritual truth that would arm me against the despair tragedy brings. I learned that even though tragedy leaves its mark on us forever, the consequences of that tragedy need not remain unchanged. I learned that if I pushed against my limits while resting in God's love, I could indeed experience the beauty of the ripples and understand the sacred truth that something remarkable is hidden in my brokenness.

This is why I can say without a doubt, *I know that something remarkable is hiding in your brokenness,* just as it was in mine. As we struggle to make sense of our pain, at first we do not know what to do; however, as we embark on this journey, God reveals the way. As we move onward each day to confront our newfound limitations and challenges, God shows us the sacred lessons that only our limitations can teach.

THE BLIND SEE, THE DEAF HEAR, AND THE LAME LEAP FOR JOY

Our limitations can either lead us to self-hatred or show us the meaning of beauty and love. The choice is ours. What our limitations and brokenness become in our lives depends on our vision. I believe there is a spiritual element to all physical acts, and the spiritual realm is accessible to all. I can't jump over a high bar like an Olympian, but the act of jumping is accessible in my heart and in my prayer life. We unleash many possibilities when we believe that this spiritual realm exists. Those who are unwilling to believe are cut off from endless possibilities. This sacred realm beyond physical reality is a place where the blind see, the deaf hear, and the lame leap for joy, even though they remain physically unable to do so. Our entering into such a sacred place— hidden deep within our inner experience and union with God—holds out for us infinite possibilities.

Let me tell you the story of a remarkable man named Jacques Lusseyran (1924–1971). Blinded in an accident when he was nearly eight years old, he learned to see with inner sight. Even though he was blind, he wrote about seeing; he did not see actual objects any longer, but he saw the world with an inner eye. During the Nazi occupation of France, he started a resistance group called the Volunteers of Liberty. In order to size up each new recruit, he would look at them through an inner eye and decide through his inner vision whether the person was sincere and worth the risk of inclusion in the group's illegal activities. Unfortunately, he made one critical misjudgment: he allowed a person into the group who was, in fact, an informant.

Lusseyran was arrested and sent to Buchenwald. At his initial interrogation, the Nazis were frustrated because they were looking for the leader hiding behind the efforts of the invalid blind man. Of course there was no one to be found, because Lusseyran himself was the group's mastermind. Obviously, because of his blindness, Lusseyran did not fit the "master race" ideal. The only reason he was allowed to live was that it was late in the war and the Nazis were no longer sure that they would win the war. Rather than deal with the consequences of putting the "invalids" to death, the Nazis formed what was known as the invalid block in each camp, and "invalids" such as Lusseyran were allowed to live. Lusseyran's experience at the invalid block was horrific: "People were dying there at a pace which made it impossible to make any count of the block. It was a greater surprise to fall over the living than the dead ... For days and nights on end, I didn't walk around, I crawled. I made an opening for myself in the mass of flesh. My hands traveled from the stump of a leg to a dead body, from the body to a wound. I could no longer hear anything for the groaning all around me."[8]

I can't imagine what Lusseyran's experience must have been like. It boggles the mind; it's beyond comprehension. I can truly say that I love

8. Jacques Lusseyran, *And There Was Light: The Autobiography of a Blind Hero of the French Resistance*, trans. Elizabeth R. Cameron (New York: Parabola, 1998) 279.

this man, even though I never met him or heard his voice. His story of survival is a masterpiece. He reached deep down into himself to find God and the truth he needed in order to endure the immense suffering of a concentration camp. During his time there, he taught his fellow prisoners about the flowing light he could see with his inner sight. He wrote, "I could try to show . . . [my fellow prisoners] how to go about holding on to life. I could turn towards them the flow of light and joy which had grown so abundant in me."[9] His fellow prisoners named him "the man who didn't die."

When I became acquainted with Lusseyran's story through his book *And There Was Light*, I had known an inner experience with God, but Lusseyran allowed me to appreciate how deep is the wellspring. He helped me know more clearly what was happening when I would enter into my inner chamber to know transformation as it comes to us from the love of God. Lusseyran offered clues about what to do with my pain when no new possibilities of assuaging it seemed to exist. He wrote of his blindness: "They told me that to be blind meant not to see. Yet how was I to believe them when I saw? Not at once, I admit . . . For at that time I still wanted to use my eyes. I followed their usual path. I looked in the direction where I was in the habit of seeing before the accident and there was anguish, a lack, something like a void which filled me with what grownups call despair."[10]

When Lusseyran looked, expecting to see with physical sight just as he did before, he fell into despair, so he struggled to look with a different pair of eyes. His inner sight emerged when he realized his eyes were not to see things as objects any longer, but as something more amazing. As Lusseyran learned to look for new possibilities, his inner vision lighted up: "I began to look more closely, not at things but at a world closer to my-self, looking from an inner place to one further within, instead of clinging to the sight toward the world outside. Immediately, the substance of the universe drew together, redefined and peopled itself anew. I was aware of a radiance emanating . . . It was a fact, for light was there."[11]

His inner sight illuminated a new dimension of existence that most never believe exists. In this second attempt at looking, Lusseyran found

9. Ibid., 282.
10. Ibid., 16.
11. Ibid., 16–17.

inner sight. How exactly did this occur? Lusseyran looked without expecting to see with physical sight. This freed him to look in a new way, and the shift in expectation allowed inner sight to come to life.

When we are broken, nothing is the same. When brokenness arrives uninvited on our doorstep, we must choose to ask ourselves, "What does it mean that I now have to live this way? What new possibilities can my new life bring?" In order to be able to dig to find it, we must believe that the hidden treasure exists. This means that we must be willing to question what we believe. Can we, within the depths of our hearts, believe that new possibilities exist, even though tragedy has struck and our lives are forever changed? Can we believe that a spiritual dimension of what we have lost exists, even though we cannot lay our hands or eyes upon it? Can we trust what our heart tells us, even though spiritual reality feels like a figment of our imagination? As we struggle to answer these questions, if we have faith, we are plunged into the depths of the inner soul.

Lusseyran shows us the way to access the spiritual dimension that lives just beyond the surface of things—and describes the drastic consequences for those who cannot venture into it:

> When I was fifteen I spent long afternoons with a blind boy my own age, one who went blind, I should add, in circumstances very like my own [—an accident]. Today I have few memories as painful. This boy terrified me. He was the living image of everything that might have happened to me if I had not been fortunate, more fortunate than he. For he was really blind. He had seen nothing since his accident. His faculties were normal, he could have seen as well as I. But they [his parents] kept him from doing so. To protect him, as they put it, they cut him off from everything, and made fun of all his attempts to explain what he felt. In grief and revenge, he had thrown himself into brutal solitude. Even his body lay prostrate in the depths of an armchair.[12]

Lusseyran's friend knows only tragedy in his brokenness and lack of sight, whereas Lusseyran finds God in his blindness through inner sight. Lusseyran believes his blindness is a blessing, but for his friend, blindness is final and unblessed. The blind lad is oblivious to the inner world that Jacques knows is real.

Lusseyran's ability to find God through inner sight is the essence of what I like to call the mystical vision. Rather than meaning by this the

12. Ibid., 31.

extraordinary experiences of God found among the saints, I mean the everyday mysticism of experiencing God's presence, a mysticism that all religious people can know and enjoy.

By contrast, when we see only tragedy in our lives, we are caught in the tragic vision, focusing primarily on the finality of what has been lost. If we dwell too much on our limitations, it is likely that we will fall into the tragic vision, and despair will result. When tragedy strikes, it is easy to fixate on our losses. As the tragic vision takes hold, it becomes increasingly difficult to listen for God and experience the love that is all around us. Anger and bitterness begin to eat away at the part of us that would seek to know God. In our pain and suffering, we become deaf to God's voice. Everywhere we look, everywhere we go, we see an endless stream of tragedy. Even if we try to forget about it for a little while, it continues to shadow us. Its contours change, yet it is endlessly with us. Consumed by our loss, the things that usually delight us no longer please us, and we begin to believe ourselves to be God's Great Victim. Anger and bitterness can gnaw at us for years and even for a lifetime, if we let them. After all, we think, this is not what my life *should* be.

When the tragic vision takes hold, the soul collapses in upon itself so that vision beyond one's own experience of tragedy becomes impossible. Thankfulness and gratitude are out of the question. There is nothing new to discover; this or that unfortunate event happened, and it is the end. The tragic vision is different from the "dark night of the soul" as described by Saint John of the Cross. In the dark night, the soul is not self-focused; rather, it seeks to find God yet experiences nothingness. Those in the midst of the dark night feel abandoned because they cannot find God, whereas those held by the tragic vision cannot seek God enough to feel abandoned. Instead, they see only the darkness, know only despair, and are unable to comprehend the potential goodness in their situations; they believe only in the finality of their own pain. We see this clearly in Jacques Lusseyran's portrayal of his friend slumping in his armchair, unable to see, whereas Jacques, though blind, sees with his inner sight.

We are called to have the same courage as Lusseyran. We are called to continue to believe in God and God's love, regardless of our suffering, pain, and brokenness. Our challenge is to resist becoming one with the darkness; instead, we are to view the darkness as only a part of life. Our encounter with darkness requires us to point ourselves in a new direction to seek life, love, and even happiness. It calls us to pierce the darkness by giving ourselves to life in spite of the pain we feel.

What does it take to move from seeing mostly darkness to experiencing the love of God? It takes keeping our hearts and minds fixed on the mystical vision. The tragic vision leads us to darkness and despair, while the mystical vision sets us on the path toward healing and transformation. The mystical vision, looking beyond the negative aspects of tragedy, finds new possibilities for hope. Those who, like Lusseyran, hold the mystical vision say to themselves, "Although I have suffered loss, the loss is not final, and it certainly does not express the essence of my life." This perspective allows us to know our suffering in a more positive way. It gives us the opportunity to find inner healing and transformation. It is not a magic formula to remove our suffering and pain. We will continue to mourn, and many more tears will fall, but the tears will have new meaning.

Seeing our current circumstances as a beginning rather than an end curtails the tragic vision and opens the way to God. As we move forward in our quest for transformation, we are challenged to shift our focus from the surface of things to a deeper, more spiritual reality. As we look into the depths with a spiritual and penetrating vision, we are likely to discover a hidden blessing in our brokenness. This blessing helps us believe that a far more beautiful life exists just beyond the horizon of our current pain. Belief in this hidden blessing is the mystical vision; and when we see with this vision, we experience the beautiful mystery of God's love.

How does the mystery of God's love reveal itself? It is hard to pinpoint what makes us able to move toward God when we are paralyzed by loss and grief. For me, God's grace works mysteriously upon my heart, and although I feel I am worthless and my life is devoid of meaning, I am somehow able to move forward toward God in prayer with hope of the fulfillment of love. We make our way toward the mystical vision through tiny steps in prayer, crying out to God wherever and whenever we feel hopeless. This translates into nearly all the time, especially when we are feeling the ill effects of the tragic vision.

When I seek a mystical vision, I pray in silent prayer. This is different than other forms of prayer where the needs of others are the focus. As I begin to pray, I close my eyes and move inward to closeout distractions. Everything calls forth within me to remain open and to try to listen for the whisper of God's love. It is frightening to open one's soul completely to God. So there are times when I have purposely turned my ears away. I press forward in silent prayer hoping for comfort and longing for love. As I reach the limits of truth that my heart and soul can know on its own. I move beyond the surface of things and into a world of the unknown. Here courage and faith are needed for I know not where the prayer will take me, for I have stepped out of myself leaving behind all my wants and desires in the hope of meeting God.

In continued silence I seek to feel the love of God. My soul questions, "If God is all Goodness, why am I left wanting for divine love?" How it is that I am to wait in this divine absence that seems endless? I am inpatient. I forget easily that it takes time to reach the divine and that on many occasions of prayer, meeting the divine simply does not happen. When my prayer meets God, my prayer longs, waits and is the fire of pure desire. The desire is a desire for an experience of God's grace that opens up the way to the mystical vision. Here I wait in silence for the touch of divine love to come and knock on the door of my heart. And to have divine love enter there in. Alas, is that a knock that I hear. Almost without notice I realize that it is no longer I alone that moves within my soul. God is with me. Yes, yes, it is true divine love is here again to greet me with its tender touch. No words are spoken here only the purity of love is exchanged and shared. Love resonates within bringing in its wake joy, tears, and sometimes pain. It is hard to feel all that love when one's soul is consumed with so many losses, so sometimes pain follows along with the touch of divine love. I experience God's love for my inner most being. The time of prayer allows me to experience life beyond my concrete concerns to enter into something much more cosmic that invites a world of possibility that without God there would be none. And what is the possibility, you ask, it is the possibility for the experience of love, goodness and healing.

Ah, how sweet is truth that comes gently, offering us words of wisdom and comfort! The words of truth are these: *Desire healing, desire love, and put your faith and trust in God; then you will find your tragic circumstances much easier to bear.*

God's love speaks to us every day through creation, but we, in our pain, are unable to hear it. Even though we cannot see, comprehend, or imagine it, the wind blows, and so God offers love to the world. In some incomprehensible way, we become aware of the faint reality of that love. We hear it over the clamor of our pain, and we see it in a few dim rays cutting through the darkness. God's love becomes more comprehensible to us as the sky, the sun, and the clouds mysteriously proclaim its reality. All nature speaks, and we hear it as love. When our eyes are not veiled, we can see the light ever so slightly peeking through the darkness. And when we can hear the joy of the birds singing their morning songs, we know we are moving closer to the mystical vision.

SWINGING

Warmth fills my body as my mother carries me into the bedroom after a bath. I feel so good. She dries me off affectionately and dresses me in my nice soft pajama top. I can't wear my pajama pants to bed tonight. The doctors say I need to wear night casts to keep my legs from bending the wrong way. So much for comfort! My mother tightens the last strap on the cast and kisses me goodnight. "Leave the light on!" I exclaim, as her hand reaches for the light switch. She blows me a kiss and then fades off into the dark hallway. I debate whether to loosen the straps and find comfort or to do what is right and suffer the pain. Some nights, I decide for comfort. When I do, my mother instinctively knows, and before she retires for the night, she creeps quietly to my bedside and does the saintly deed of putting the casts back on me. Saintly, because she is inflicting pain with a holy purpose.

As I try to fall asleep, I look at the circle of light the lamp reflects on the ceiling. "God," I begin to pray, "I want to run and play like the other children. Why can't I? I will try harder, and perhaps tomorrow, you will make me well. I love you, God. Thanks for having fun with me on the swing today." My time on the swing earlier that day would mark the beginning of knowing God powerfully as the One who lives intimately in my soul.

~

I lay my crutches in the long grass of the side yard. As I move, I lean on the plastic riding horse to maintain my balance. I ride the horse often. I hop on it and push down on the pedals, and the horse moves back and forth. From the horse, I watch my siblings pump the swings and move so high in the air. I dream that I too will touch the sky. Next to them, I ride my horse as my imagination carries me off into the sunset. The horse has never allowed me to touch the sky like my siblings can.

With one hand on the plastic horse's mane, I resolve: "This will be the day that I touch the sky." I push off the horse and speedily grab the chain on one side of the swing. As quickly as I can, I pivot around to take hold of the second chain, and now the seat of the swing is beneath me. I can't jump up on the swing, so I take two or three careful steps back to get the seat squarely against my bottom. When I do this, I know it is time to pull myself up quickly with my arms (made strong from my crutches), so my feet no longer touch the ground. In one motion I sit and let the swing take me.

I have done this before. The swing always moves me a few times back and forth before the motion begins to fade. I instinctively stand up when the swing stops and follow the same procedure of stepping back and hoisting myself back up onto the seat. I glide some more until the swing stops again. This is how I swing day after day.

Today is different. Today I am going to touch the sky. Instead of hopping off the swing when it stops, I sit still, carefully balancing. Amazed, I realize how different it feels to balance on the swing, motionless. I hang onto the chains that support me now much as my crutches do. I try to visualize how my siblings touch the sky. Mimicking their motions, I lean back as my legs instinctively move out straight. The swing moves forward and I say to myself, "Wow, I moved the swing!"

Startled by the movement, I bend my arms, pushing myself forward while my legs remain straight. The spasticity of my cerebral palsy demands this. I close my eyes and again see my siblings riding way up high with their legs bent under the swing. "Bend your knees!" I order. "Bend your knees! God, please help me bend," I pray. "Please help me bend, please help me bend."

I swing several times with my legs remaining straight and my arms working extra hard to perpetuate movement. I am pleased that I am moving the swing. The joy of the movement fills me and I begin to sing, "O Lord, you are God, and you love me." The sun beams down on the trees, making the sky look fresh—crisp and extra blue with soft, white, fluffy clouds. The birds hear my song and add their own version. I think if I can just touch the treetops, God will be there.

The swing stops as my arms get tired, and when I finish my one-line song to God, I whisper to myself, as everything feels undeniably sacred, "Just relax and bend." My entire being continues with the song, "O Lord, you are God, and you love me." I lean back straight, and then forward, and bend; back and straight, forward, and bend; and now I am moving closer and closer to the sky. Upward, upward, closer to God I go.

Now I swing out and up into the open arms. My song is louder and more robust. The wind rushes through the three great big maple trees. I watch them move closer and then farther away as I hear the swing creak against its hooks. The sun dances and shifts its light on the leaves as the wind plays with them. Through the movement back and forth, God touches my soul. All the creatures in nature invite me to know the truth of their origin in God. The trees, grass, sky, birds, and clouds speak to me in unison as I reach for the treetops and sky with my newfound freedom on the swing. Suddenly, the truth I have been singing springs into life in my very soul: "O Lord, you are God, and you love me."

Bursting forth, God's love knows me, touches me, and searches the depths of my heart. I sing to God, God hears me, and I feel God's love all the more intensely. Nothing can break the intimacy between the creature and the Creator. Up high, oh way up high, I feel union with God as I try to touch the sky. I know I am who I am truly meant to be. And forevermore, I resolve to seek God's presence again and again. Reaching both forward and back in time, somehow my little heart knows that a battle lies ahead, and this day I know that God will be with me every step of the way. Love moves the consuming difficulty of disability far into the distance as freedom gives me a song to sing.

My childhood commitment to knowing and loving God set the stage for further moments of openness, for more experiences of the mystical vision. When we are open to God, we are open to all the emerging possibilities life has to offer. We are in the swing and; we are on the pool's edge. No matter the height of our ride or the breadth of our splash, we have put ourselves where miracles can happen, and that is a prerequisite to receiving them. The mystical vision begins by believing in the possibilities hidden in opportunities. My opportunity came while I was on the swing. I could have sat on my horse, sobbing the hours away. Thank God, I wanted something else to happen; I wanted to touch the sky. I was open to God, open to possibility. I accepted the opportunity to try.

The mystical vision, our new way of living, comes from being open to discover the goodness of God that lies just beyond the tragic vision. If we sort reality into neat little categories by predicting that the future will be exactly like the past, we will never transform our pain. By attending to what is good in our lives even while we are in great pain, we find that when we are ready and it is time, our perspective will change.

We may be angry at God over our tragic circumstances; or we may be depressed like Lusseyran's friend slumping in his armchair. When we get trapped in our image of what our lives should be, there is only one way to free ourselves: abandon what we once wanted for ourselves and turn to God. How can we let go of what we think should have been and accept what we now have? Our freedom to respond to events, tragic or otherwise, can never be taken from us. Viktor Frankl reminds us of this truth in his book *Man's Search for Meaning*. Frankl, who spent three years in Auschwitz, writes: "We who lived in concentration camps can remember the men who walked through the huts, comforting others, giving away their last piece of bread. They may have been few in number, but they offer sufficient proof that everything can be taken from a man but one thing: the last of human freedoms—to choose one's attitude in any given set of circumstances, to choose one's own way."[13]

We have the power to choose our response to tragic circumstances. And if we believe in God, we realize that we don't have to choose our attitude on our own. God is with us. In fact, if we try to go it alone, we are likely to fail. Our helper is God, the Almighty, the Holy One of Israel. God seeks to be with us in our pain. However, to let God in, we must let go of the life we once thought we should have had. Letting go does not mean that we have to enjoy everything about our life as it is. We simply must be willing to turn away from the past that "should have been" and to look forward to future opportunities.

I know it may feel impossible to look forward, and the pain can feel unbearable. Lusseyran tells us that the best and most certain remedy for our suffering is to focus completely and unreservedly on the present moment. He writes:

"Latch on to the passing minute. Shut off the workings of memory and hope. The amazing thing is that no anguish held out against this treatment lasts for very long. Take away from suffering its double drumbeat of resonance, memory and fear. Suffering may persist, but already it is relieved by half. Throw yourself into each moment as if it were the only one that really existed. Work and work hard."[14]

13. Viktor E. Frankl, *Man's Search for Meaning* (New York: Pocket, 1963) 104.

14. Lusseyran, *And There Was Light*, 290.

Focusing on the present moment kept Lusseyran alive in the concentration camp. As we take Lusseyran's advice, our focus shifts from the life we thought we should have had to the life we have now. We detach ourselves from our desire for a different set of circumstances. Even when our hearts cry out, "I don't want to endure any longer if this is how it is going to be!" we learn to surrender ourselves to this moment and the next. As we let go of our desires, we are able to let God into the present moment.

It is not always easy to accept our circumstances, even one moment at a time, but this is indeed what we must try to do. Each new gesture toward acceptance moves us closer to God. As we string more of these moments of acceptance together, we find that we are no longer trapped by the feelings of despair that held us captive day after day. If we find we can't give all our pain to God, we must do the next best thing and give God what we can. God will take whatever we can give when we say, "Here you go: it's yours. I don't like it. I don't understand it. I put my tragic circumstances in your hands."

When we are willing to accept our situation unconditionally, we unleash untold possibilities. Make no mistake about it: the impossible becomes possible only with God. Possibility as God conceives it may not always match our concept of what it should be, but it exists as abundant potential just the same. Hidden in our brokenness is the promise of experiencing love and knowing God. When we see the possibilities that life offers us, God invites us to act upon those possibilities in faith.

When we accept our brokenness, our fractured lives are no longer an avenue for pain, but something far more remarkable—a conduit for intimacy with God. And if we are willing to venture into the depths of our pain to act faithfully, God teaches us the divine lessons that grow through the cracks of our fragmented beings and bodies. Intimacy flourishes and knowledge abounds when we are willing to live with our pain, knowing that God is ready to teach us these sacred truths. Reaching into the depths of our souls through prayer and attention, we meet the divine mystery who provides us with the beginning of the spiritual knowledge that transforms our suffering. Our mystical vision strengthens our union with God.

THREE

Along the Way with the Mystical Vision and a Supportive Community

THE MYSTICAL VISION SETS us free. When we have it, suffering is not the last word; rather, we see the beauty in all of life and believe in the dawning of love just beyond the darkness. Life is not a prison where suffering holds us captive; rather, it is an adventure to a better kind of life. Moments of despair and discouragement do not linger, because we are ever searching for the way to set the swing in motion once more. All-encompassing goodness surrounds us, transforming reality into new and ever-expanding possibilities. When goodness breaks through the darkness, when we reach for the skies with our toes again, we encounter the love of God.

The mystical vision does not come to us magically. It comes through quieting ourselves from within so that we can know God in our pain. It comes from lessons learned along the way on our healing journey. Some people live their entire lives unable to recognize the goodness that envelops them. If we are to see and understand, we must develop prayerful attention.

Prayerful attention is different from the prayers we say on behalf of others or in church services. It means listening intently for God, which initiates the process of inner healing. It means shifting our attention from what is concretely in front of us to what is hidden in the spiritual realm. It means taking the time to look.

PRAYERFUL ATTENTION

Guigo, a twelfth-century monk, wrote, "Prayer is the heart's devoted turning to God to drive away evil and obtain what is good."[1] Although tragedy

1. Guigo II, *The Ladder of Monks: A Letter on the Contemplative Life and Twelve*

is not synonymous with evil, we are wise to consider Guigo's perspective on prayer. When we engage in prayerful attention, we make a parallel shift: we focus our attention on God, turning away from the tragedy that has hit us.

Refocusing our attention is not easy. Our pain is real and strong—are we to employ heroic tactics and deny it? No, we are not in denial when we turn our focus on God. Rather, we reach a deeper level of awareness when we see the potential goodness that can live within tragedy and brokenness. Lusseyran shows us that attention opens up the way for transformation. Our beloved blind friend explains that, "Being attentive unlocks a sphere of reality that no one suspects. If, for instance, I walked along the path without being attentive, completely immersed in myself, I did not know whether trees grew along the way, nor how tall they were, or whether they had leaves. When awakened with attention, however, every tree immediately came to me."[2]

It is not just the act of attention itself, but the specific form of attention, that is important. Only attention immersed in prayer will make the mystical vision present to us, opening up a new dimension of reality immersed in mystery. Prayerful attention gives us radical new insight as we quiet our hearts and focus our minds in order to open ourselves to God. As Lusseyran discovered, "The shadow of a tree on the road is not only a visual phenomenon. It is also audible."[3]

Prayer brings us beyond the difficulty of not being able to do what we want when we want to; it brings us into the presence of God, who provides us with consolation and courage to live beyond our suffering for another day. To move past brokenness, we must encounter God in an inner chamber that many do not know exists. The poet-theologian Ernesto Cardenal writes that, "Everyone has an inner room. Deep inside every human being there is a nuptial chamber where only the bridegroom comes. We all have within us a dark secret place, a locked room, created for love, an inner paradise. But most people do not know it is there."[4] As a

---

Meditations, trans. Edmund Colledge and James Walsh, Cistercian Studies Series 48 (Kalamazoo, MI: Cistercian, 1979) 68.

2. Jacques Lusseyran, *Against the Pollution of the I: Selected Writings* (New York: Parabola, 1999) 32.

3. Ibid., 65.

4. Ernesto Cardenal, *Love: A Glimpse of Eternity*, rev. ed. (Brewster, MA: Paraclete, 2006; orig. ed. 1970) 51.

Christian, Cardenal is speaking of Christ, the bridegroom. For a Jew, this would be similar to the Shekhinah, or divine immanence. Whatever our faith community, it is in our inner room, through prayer, that we are most likely to find God.

Prayer is not always about words. We may not have words for God when tragedy takes hold, but God is waiting to meet us in our pain. When we step back from our restlessness and our hearts become quiet, we come to know the truth that God lives with us. God greets us every day no matter what the day brings. With infinite love and wisdom, God holds us, giving us strength and courage to go about our business for another day in spite of our frustration and discouragement.

So here's the call to you, my friend: if you are in pain on this very day, let God in. Find a quiet, comfortable place and rest awhile, leaving the world and your problems behind. Take one deep breath and then another. Close your eyes and let God in to hold you and touch you and reveal a holy presence to your soul.

I have to be truthful: this prayerful time will not wipe away your pain. But your soul will know the consolation of God, and that is a promise. If you accept this consolation, it will bring you much happiness and joy even in your pain. Let it all go; let your pain fall into the arms of God. Let your soul relax and rest itself in God. Let the awareness of God come, and when it does, you enter your inner world. This awareness does not prompt you to give a litany of petitions; here you are not overwhelmed by your smallness in relation to your Creator. Instead, you sense God's loving hand holding you and giving you peace. In this inner place, the divine presence touches your deepest need. You move beyond the world of appearances and the concrete situation of brokenness to a spiritual reality. In your inner world, you find God's love.

You know that you are beginning to make the connection when the storm winds of tragedy threaten to blow you away and you decide not to succumb to them. Instead, you move against the wind. Leaning forward into the storm, you resolve to know God, and God greets you from within. At first you may feel overwhelmed by God's presence, but you quickly realize that God wants to share intimate moments with you, to call you into deep spiritual insight and knowledge that builds trust and faith in God. This realization came to me when I was learning to walk for the doctors at Children's Hospital.

WALKING AT CHILDREN'S HOSPITAL

I walk for the doctors at Children's Hospital wearing just my underwear. At the age of five, I am unembarrassed about my bare body. The lack of clothing serves an important purpose: my near nakedness allows the doctors to see my hips jut out awkwardly from side to side with my every step. As I teeter across the examination room, my bare feet slap the shiny black linoleum floor. My feet can't do the normal heel-toe motion; at best, they hit the floor squarely with a slap. I hate the slapping sound because it reminds me that I am not normal like my brothers and sisters, and normal is exactly what I long to be. Every slap reminds me that I am not who I would like to be.

But that aside, these moments of walking make me happy because I am doing something I love—walking without my crutches and braces. It feels good to be unshackled from all that metal and wood. I want to walk perfectly now to show the doctors and my mother that I don't need any of that. To banish my crutches and braces forever—that is my goal. Several times a day, my mother asks me, "Where are your crutches?" My crutches usually are in the bushes, on the sidewalk, or in the backyard—anywhere they won't be used.

I hear the doctors talking medical gibberish. I look at my mother watching me from her chair, her bleached-blond beehive hairdo riding high in the air. Putting her elbow on her crossed leg and her hand under her chin, she settles in for the unfolding drama of my careful steps. She must think, "How far we have come—but how much further do we have to go?" She tries to understand everything that is happening; she doesn't want the doctors to pull one over on us.

Because I am her precious project, she demands not only my best but the impossible. She helps me believe that one day I will be able to do anything I want to do. I will run marathons; I will leap tall buildings in a single bound. Whenever the doctors tell my mother "She won't be able to," we both take notice and get busy. We will push and push against this cerebral palsy until it breaks. All that pushing means hours and hours of physical therapy on our own, day after day. If the sheet of stick figures describing my physical-therapy exercises says two times daily for five days a week, to us that really meant three times daily for seven days a week. My mother and I want to achieve perfection. We plan to teach all those bright,

Harvard-educated doctors that they don't know everything, and that they certainly are unqualified to make predictions about my life.

To take that perfect step—that is my wish. To move the "right" way, just like everyone else. "Yes, yes, just that way," I say to myself as I step forward. In my mind's eye I see how my siblings walk. Now it's my turn. I step again, and the voices of the doctors and my mother fade as I descend into my inner world. In my depths, I know God as a miraculous, warm white light. Here God helps me walk. God does not demand perfection, even though that is what I seek. Instead, the warm white light sends a quiet feeling of love throughout my body that asks me to respond, using my inner world. I reach down, down, further down, into the love that lives inside. My mind pulls everything from within to make the steps happen. Now step, heel toe, watch your arms, right-arm-left foot, left-arm-right-foot. Let's try to get those heels down, one and two. Keep trying. Don't give up.

I talk to myself, but now I know I am walking under the power of God. The sacred drama shared with God brings knowledge of the truth: I am no longer a crippled little girl; I am the one who can move mountains, even the mountain of cerebral palsy. This faith, a gift from God, comes to me in waves as I take my twenty paces to the other side of the room and back again. I know that I am capable. "Touch your nose with your toes," my mother says during our physical-therapy sessions to help me get my heels to touch the floor first. I think of this now as I press on. "Ah, there's a heel, do you see that? I had a heel right there, three paces ago. Are you guys looking?" I yell in my mind. I know that my private victory does not go unnoticed. God sees.

The mountain of my cerebral palsy breaks free from its moorings. My feet continue to slap, but what a beautiful slapping it is. For if they were not slapping, they would be dragging; and if not dragging, crawling—and if not crawling, not moving at all. The slapping is on the outside, but on the inside, my movements are transformed into a dance with God. There is more to a miracle than what meets the eye. Even though the doctors see my body as convoluted, distorted, and broken, I know that something else is true. I know my body is loved. My foot-slapping gait brings me to an intimate dance with the Creator, whose mystical power brings good from evil and transforms my suffering into new life.

The doctors cannot see what lies beyond my distorted movements. They want me to perform the "normal" way. They are blind to the beauty and love surrounding my encounter with God, because they see my walking only with the naked eye. The doctors fail to see that my unsightly brokenness actually leads me to experience God's holiness.

Truly I found inner healing that day. Inner healing requires venturing beyond our painful, concrete reality into an inner reality that provides peace and consolation. When we enter into this inner reality, we travel through our pain to find love. Courage helps us see beyond the darkness, and hope puts an endless array of possibilities before us. Then, undaunted by the obstacles in our path, we are able to step out in faith.

Through faith Lusseyran survived the camp, and Carretto remained in the desert. Through faith my mother held herself steady, allowing me to have as normal a childhood as possible. Through faith I heard God's call to look deeply within myself as I tried to make my steps happen at Children's Hospital. Through faith I said to the mountain of my cerebral palsy, "Be lifted up and thrown into the sea" (Matthew 21:21). I answered God's call through prayerful attention and thoughtful action. Over and over again during my childhood, God would ask me to respond to new challenges, and I would struggle to carry on in faithfulness.

FAITHFULNESS

It takes faith to identify and act on the possibilities revealed by our mystical vision. When Jesus' disciples wondered why they could not cure a boy with epilepsy, he told them it was "Because of your little faith. For truly I tell you, if you have faith the size of a mustard seed, you will say to this mountain, 'Move from here to there,' and it will move, and nothing will be impossible for you" (Matthew 17:20).

Faith is fundamental to Jesus' teaching. Over and over again, in all four Gospels, Jesus encourages people to come to him in faith. We can read his words about the immense power of faith—the power to move trees and even mountains—in Matthew 17 and 21, Mark 11, and Luke 17. And this mighty faith need only be the size of a tiny mustard seed.

When I was young, I constantly asked God for a miracle: "God, I want to be normal. I want to walk and be like all my siblings." I wanted God to wave a magic wand at my command and grant my wish. It's not uncommon for people to think that if God is the Creator of the universe, of course he will give us what we want . . . even if it means defying the natural laws of the universe. (Imagine saying to that tree hanging just over your neighbor's property, "Hey, you tree in my front yard, move a few feet to the right, would you please?") In the Scriptures, we read of Jesus walking on water and healing many with a mere word or touch. And if these stories are true, or if we believe that God is a God of miracles, what does it mean that we seek with our entire being for our brokenness to be taken from us, and yet it remains? What does it mean that we cannot say to the mountain of our pain, "Be lifted up and thrown into the sea?"

Thomas Merton (1915–1968), a Christian monk, was a hermit, theologian, writer, and poet. Like Carretto and Lusseyran, he stirred in my heart and imagination for many years. I first fell in love with Merton when I read his book *The New Seeds of Contemplation*. In it, he describes in poetic meditations how to live a life of prayer. The book created in me an insatiable thirst for God, a longing for intimacy with God beyond all else. I wanted more God, more love, and much more time for prayer. This, of course, inspired me to read more of Merton's books, and in his words I found explanations about the life of faith that I carry in my heart wherever I go. One of these explanations helped me understand mountain-moving faith. Merton writes:

> When we read in the New Testament of faith "moving mountains" we must not interpret the symbolic language in an exclusively literal sense, as if it meant that prayer were a wonderful means of accomplishing physically difficult or impossible tasks. This is the kind of inanity that atheists come up with, after they have moved a hill with a bulldozer ... Faith does indeed deal with impossibilities: but it is not intended as a substitute for mere physical power, or medicine, or study, or human investigation.
>
> When Christ taught his hearers that they must have faith, he did not intend that they merely should use it to change the landscape. He was telling men their faith should be of a kind that was not daunted by any obstacle or any apparent impossibility. The lesson was directed to the qualities of faith, not to the nature of the task to be done. The task did not matter, because *anything* that was necessary for salvation would be granted by God in answer to prayer.[5]

When I consider this text, I imagine myself with a wheelbarrow, a pick, and a shovel, working really hard at digging out a gigantic mountain. Sweating, I repeat my mantra: "This is the faith that moves mountains.

5. Thomas Merton, *Life and Holiness* (New York: Image, 1963) 81–82.

This is the faith that moves mountains." I get only so far in my imagination before I think, "I really do need a bulldozer."

Even though my fantasy focuses on the task (and that's what Merton is trying to deemphasize), I quickly see that mountain-moving faith isn't about geological engineering. Rather, it is about being undaunted by the apparent impossibility of what I am being asked to do. When life hands us brokenness, it is as if God says to us, "Here is your mountain. Your faith will move it." As Merton reminds us, faith is not waving a magic wand and making the mountain move, but rather being undaunted by the prospect of having to dig through what our brokenness asks of us every day.

Faith sets us on the path to healing. As we continue the journey, we grow in love and intimacy with God. Love fills us with the courage to hope, and hope pushes us to accomplish the next task God is calling us to do.

SKATING

In faith, my mother gave me a pair of "double runners"—ice skates with four blades—when I was six years old. They strapped onto my shoes like a pair of old-fashioned roller skates, the extra blades steadying them just as training wheels steady a bike. Every day after school, much to my delight, I would abandon my crutches and my braces for my special skates and try to be just like my brothers and sisters. To be like all the other children in my family and the neighborhood was my secret wish. Every night before going to sleep I would pray, "God, please make it so I can play like all the other children."

For me it was a long, difficult trek across our snow-covered backyard to the vacant lot just behind our house, where my father had set up a homemade ice rink just for us. When I got there, I would crawl around on the ice trying to stand up until I got tired. Then I would play in the snow as I watched my brothers and sisters play hockey. At the end of each day my brother Joe would stand me up so I could feel what it was like to be upright on the ice. Soon my legs would slip out from under me, and Joe would gently lower me back into a sitting position. He would skate away from me in silence so I could experience my pain alone.

Then one sunny Sunday afternoon it happened: my brother stood me up—and I kept standing. Amazed, he skated backward away from me to see if I could continue to stand independently, and I did. He called out,

"Skate to me, Diana," and I did. He ran off into the snow with his skates on, leaving me standing in the middle of the ice. He screamed for our parents, who were in the house, "Come see, Diana is skating!"

Our parents rushed to the second-floor window to watch. The hockey game stopped immediately, and everyone looked at me in disbelief. There was a strange silence, and then my sister Mariann said, "Skate, Diana, skate!" I skated awkwardly, of course, but the sun was shining, the kids were all out playing, and for once I was one of them. God had answered my prayer! It was a miracle. For once, I felt normal. I thought I had crossed the barrier separating me from the other kids, never to fall back into my old disabled ways.

The next day, I could not wait to come home from school and be normal again. I wanted to again abandon my crutches and braces and go to the magical place on the ice with my special skates. But when I tried to stand, my legs slipped out from under me and down I went. I tried and tried, to no avail. No more miracles—God was fresh out. The ice was hard, and the sun was not shining.

It hurt. I cried. But I felt oddly thankful, too, because even as a little girl, I knew how wonderful it had been to have my day, to have my miracle. It is natural to want our miracles and encounters with God to come on our own terms; we want God to have that magic wand ready and working on our behalf. It is easier to act faithfully when we believe the miracle we want, just the way we want it, is lying just beyond our reach. But our ways are not God's ways, and our notions of healing and miracles are not God's.

Edith Barfoot (1887–1975) suffered most of her life with crippling arthritis. Bedridden for nearly eighty years, she could have allowed her unfortunate situation to rob her of her faith in God. After all, how could a loving God permit such pain to overtake her entire body? Instead, she allowed her suffering to lead her deeper into belief that God is love, and she experienced love for God in the midst of her suffering and brokenness. She wrote that, "The soul must ever remember that he who calls for her response is God her Father, and that always it is the call of Love, no matter how much hardness and difficulty the call might hold for her. Deep down in the soul of every child of his there is the longing to be called by our Father to do something special for him."[6]

6 Edith Barfoot, *The Witness of Edith Barfoot: The Joyful Vocation to Suffering* (Oxford: Blackwell, 1977; orig. ed. 1957) 1.

The special thing that Edith Barfoot did for God was to lie in bed for years, wracked with pain, solely to bear testimony to God's loving care and call upon her life. Her story makes us wonder: what gave her the power to accept her life so unconditionally even in her suffering? When we try to understand why one comes to believe and another does not, we move beyond the realm of factual answers, such as one and one equals two, and into the realm of mystery. The truth of God's love mysteriously revealed itself to her, and, like Lusseyran and Carretto, she listened to God's call and responded in faith.

The journey to healing always begins with a reordering of our inner world. True healing happens when a person's faith meets God's love, creating a sacred interaction that changes us inside. It is difficult to respond faithfully to God when we are in pain, and yet Edith did so with surprising ease. Her challenge to us is clear: when God calls to us in our pain, may we faithfully answer the call. And in answering, may we have courage and strength to set aside our own notions of what our healing should be, in order to follow the path God is setting before us. Let us now reshape our inner worlds by giving up our preconceived notions of what our healing should be, as we let God penetrate our inner souls with a healing touch.

My mother could have decided it was inappropriate to buy me those special skates. My brother could have decided it was pointless to help me stand on the ice. And I could have decided to give up. Instead, we all decided to have faith and to keep the way open to a miracle. If we think a miracle has happened only when an affliction is completely removed, we fail to know the miracle of God that is found in brokenness. When my mother and Joe decided to help me skate, they gave me a gift, even if it was just for one day. Each day as we faithfully worked on making my dream a reality, I wished to be able to skate every day just like my siblings. Instead, I got my one sunny day to skate. Truly a miracle found me on that day, and my soul faithfully knew it as such.

RIDING TO FREEDOM

When I was ten, I was dismayed to see my five-year-old sister, Edie, riding up and down and all around our deadend street on a bike without training wheels, her long, straight blond hair blowing in the wind. Starting at the first hill where the street intersected the main road, she would whiz by our large white house on the right to the valley past our driveway. Then she would rise from her seat and push the pedals hard to make it up the second hill. At its summit, she would spin once or twice around the large cul-de-sac we called the circle before beginning her descent down the second hill. We didn't have to worry about cars on our safe dead-end street, so the hills became the playground of all the kids in the neighborhood. I would watch the other children whizzing up and down the hills and around the circle, privately disgusted with myself for still riding a bike with training wheels—especially now that even Edie no longer needed them.

So, resolving to show Edie and my other family members a thing or two, I put the wrench on the nut and turned. The bolt and the nut attached to it turned along with the wrench. I grabbed another wrench to hold the nut while I loosened the bolt with the first wrench. The nut came off and I pulled the training wheel off. The kickstand kept the bike from falling as I asked myself, "Are you ready for this? Are you ready to ride?" I kept questioning my actions as I repeated the process on the other side of the bike. I reapplied the nuts to their respective bolts and stood up, swinging the bike from side to side, thinking, "Now there are no training wheels. My bike is free."

Anticipation and fear filled me as I walked the bike to the top of the hill just before the circle. I thought, "I will show them I can ride this bike without training wheels. I am ten, and Edie is only five. I will show them!" I mounted the bike and said aloud, "God help me." My legs pointed outward, not reaching or touching the pedals on either side. I swerved sharply to the right and then to the left as I began screaming, "God, what am I doing?" Swerving from one side to the other, I reached the valley between the hills. The bike lost momentum and I went down. I quickly got up, laughing nervously and saying, "That was great, now let's do it again." This time I started about halfway up the hill and then tumbled down.

Over and over I went up the hill, climbed on the bike, and soon fell off. Each ride down the hill would yield a different result. I would reach one pedal and not the other, or I would turn the handlebars too hard to the right or to the left. Each time I said to myself, "That was good; let's try it again." Even as the falls continued, I came closer to balancing on the two wheels. Day after day, I worked on riding my bike until I was too tired to continue. Every day God heard the same mantra from me, "Someday God, someday, please."

After each try, the vision of riding off into the sunset grew stronger. I dreamed of that summer morning or evening when I would make it down the hill without falling, my feet on the pedals and my hands holding the handlebars straight. I would soar up the hill to the intersection and glide all around the neighborhood just like my siblings. In my mind, I could see the wind in my own hair as I pedaled effortlessly up and down the sidewalks and driveways, even riding standing up for hours. One day it would happen, and my family and the neighborhood kids would see what I could do. One day I would ride just like them.

Instead of sitting around sulking over the fact that I couldn't ride a bike without training wheels, I saw another future just beyond my limited horizon. In hope, I saw the glorious possibilities; and in faith, I heard and answered God's call to take action. And that is how I moved that particular mountain.

Few neighbors dared interfere with my sacred quest. Most seemed to understand that God and I were hard at work, making a miracle happen. The other neighborhood children mostly stayed away from me. If someone tried to rescue or help me, I would yield the street to them and quickly walk my bike home to begin my quest on another day, perhaps in the quiet of the morning when I would not be disturbed. However, some nervous neighbors called my mother demanding that she take the bike away from me, and one neighbor even threatened to call Child Protective Services. My mother's reply went something like this: "For God's sake, I'm not pushing her down the hill. Do what I do—go into your house, shut your blinds, and don't watch." She always put on this brave aura, but she confessed to a friend one day that she spent a great deal of time peeking through the blinds with tears in her eyes and fear in her heart.

I think my mother knew any effort to take away my bike would have been futile. I would have taken one of my siblings' bikes or pitched such a constant fit that she would have had no choice but to give in to my longing. Up to that point, my mother had never used the word "can't" in reference to anything I wanted to do. To take away the bike would have violated her commitment to me. I think she realized that something sacred and beautiful was in the making out there on the street, and she would not be the one to end it. She let me follow my dreams in spite of persistent neighborly anxieties.

One morning as the sun had just found its way over the treetops in our neighborhood, I took my bike out for another day on the sacred playground of my street. "I know I can do this someday. Maybe this will be the day," I said to myself as I walked the bike to the spot that I had determined, after a few weeks of practice, provided me with just the right momentum to allow me to catch the pedals and even land without too much harm. Mounting the bike partway down the second hill, with the circle behind me, I said to God (as I often did during my practice sessions), "Please, God, let this be the day."

This time I pushed off the hill a little harder than usual. "Here we go," I said. "Got one pedal, oh, there's the next. Keep your head up. Handlebars steady. Haven't made it over the valley yet. Turn the pedals; keep your feet on them. Turn the pedals; do it again, again; one more time, and we are on our way up the hill. Keep going. One time around with those pedals, then another, and another, and on the way up the hill. Wow, I am going up the hill. Up, up. Here I am." Halfway up the first hill, I turned the handlebars quickly and crashed to the ground as if I were sliding into second base. I jumped for joy, saying, "God, yes! God, yes!"

I mounted the bike facing the other way, and the cul-de-sac was in front of me now. Off I went down the first hill and up the second hill and around the circle and down the hill, past my original starting place and up the first hill as far as my house. I parked my bike on the sidewalk so I could run into the house to get my mother's attention. "Look, Mom, no training wheels!" I said, pointing at the bike through the picture window in our living room, and my mother said, "Yes, Diana, I saw you. I saw you. Go ride, and have fun."

My vigilant mother had witnessed my wonderful ride. As the weeks and months continued, the worried neighbors had to relent. I was filled with joy as I rode around the neighborhood during those happy days of summer. My mother could have said, "No, no, Diana, you can't ride a bike without training wheels," and worse yet, I could have believed her. If the potential harm outweighed the benefits, of course, I would have had to endure the horror of a bikeless childhood. But I suspect my mother had faith in my ability to know my limitations better than anyone else could, so what would have been the point of closing off possibilities? Respecting my dignity and my desires, she said to the world around her, "My daughter will live in a world without limits, a place of endless possibilities." Thank God for those possibilities, and for the wonder of becoming freer every day.

Every day as I took my bike and put myself through my paces, I was being called to keep trying, called to find God in the daily disappointments and discouragement, called to look beyond the seemingly hopeless situation to a tomorrow that promised, "Yes, someday—and maybe today will be the day." I could love the long, slow process because of the wonder of my dream.

~

You may be saying to yourself, how can a child carry such passion for her dreams?

My mother taught me from a young age, "No one is going to hand you anything. If you want to, you will, and if you say you can't, you won't." If I wanted to ride, I had to be willing to go out, say my prayers, and move the mountain faithfully and in love, piece by piece. It was as if with each attempt I was taking another shovelful of dirt and casting it aside so that one day I could say, "Oh! You mountain, now that you are turned into a little mound, be cast into the sea!"

Hope sees possibilities, faith hears the call to act, and infinite love gives us the power to do so. Somehow faith, hope and love worked together to give form to the miracles of my early childhood. Hope called out to me to look and see a future without training wheels. Faith called out to me and said, "Ride, Diana, ride! Believe and know it can be true." And love inspired my inner being to do whatever it would take to make the dream become a reality.

Faith opens up the way for us to love not only the dream but also the effort required to make it come true—paying attention to every detail on the way to that perfect outcome; pushing ourselves to the limit, knowing that God is by our side through every little disappointment and in every triumph. When we approach our dreams with such faithfulness and love, the process of meeting God in our dreams means as much as or even more than crossing that sacred finish line and attaining our long-awaited desire. When I found my way to freedom on my bike, I was in love with the process and in love with God.

When we act in faith in spite of our brokenness, the people close to us can either hinder us or help us. It takes a community joining with us to nurture in us all the faithfulness and love necessary to keep our dreams alive and help them grow. Blessings of my community, my family, and all the neighborhood kids who made room for me in their childhood games, even when it was inconvenient.

NEIGHBORHOOD WIFFLE BALL

When Carlton (Pudge) Fisk entered the Baseball Hall of Fame, a part of me felt like a Hall of Famer as well. As a ten-year-old girl, I was nick-named Pudge during neighborhood games of Wiffle ball. Though Fisk was called Pudge in grade school because he was pudgy, I was not. I was given the nickname simply because I, like Fisk, was a catcher. We all took the personas of 1975 Boston Red Sox players that year. The right fielder, for example, was known as Evans for the Sox's great right fielder Dwight Evans.

The large cul-de-sac at the end of our street provided the perfect landscape for a neighborhood park. The sidewalk corners were used to mark out first and third base, while someone's jacket, hat, or other mis-cellaneous item (unknown to our mothers) became second base in the middle of the turnaround circle. Just beyond second base, we left four or five feet for an outfield. If the ball landed in a neighbor's yard behind the circle at the end of the outfield, it was a home run. At the beginning of the circle, right at the crest of the second hill, we put home plate. The catcher's job was to prevent balls from going down the hill into the valley.

On either side of the valley were two sewer drains with open-hole grates for covers. The holes were safe for our Wiffle balls, but a tennis ball could easily fit through them. If we were playing with a tennis ball—as we often did—and it got past me, one of the other children would run quickly to catch it before it went down one of those holes and subsequently ended the game. We knew we were having a bad day when we watched our ball bounce several times along the outer rim before plunging through one of the holes into the drain. Sometimes we were lucky, and one of the kids would pull another ball out of his pocket so the game could resume.

On days when there were enough players, the kids would place a backup catcher behind me just in case I missed the ball and it started toward the sewer. They had tried me in this backup position, but I could not run fast enough. Most days, I was allowed to play. When I caught, I caught for both sides, and the kids made a no-stealing rule. They knew that my crutches lay a few feet away on the sidewalk, and they couldn't justify trying to steal bases against me (although part of me secretly likes to believe that they didn't want to take the chance!)

Some days, however, the game took on a seriousness that could not tolerate a backup catcher and a no-stealing rule. On one of these days when I was not allowed to play, I began crying out, "Equal rights, equal rights!"

My mother stepped out of our front door onto the porch. She yelled up to me, "I'll equal-rights you! You get in this house right now!" The game continued without stopping for even a moment, but the kids must have felt something. A few days later, I would be laying aside my crutches and catching the ball behind home plate again, trying my best to be like the other children.

My six—at the time—siblings were friends with nearly all the other neighborhood kids, and the way my brothers and sisters treated me was the way the other kids were expected to treat me too. They did not make fun of me, they never used the derogatory word *cripple*, and they gave me the same respect any other kid could expect. They appreciated my bodily control and athletic ability, and I was happy that their nickname for me associated me with the great Carlton Fisk.

I had a Hall of Fame day myself at the end of that summer when I was ten. One cloudy August day, the neighborhood kids were sitting around our backyard with not much to do. My brother Joe and his fourteen-year-old friends thought they were beyond the pickup game of Wiffle Ball. Yet that day everyone decided to join the summer's last game.

We rode our bikes—mine without training wheels!—to the top of the hill and took our respective positions: first base by the curb, second base in the middle, third base by the opposite curb. Joe pitched; I caught the ball and threw it back. The batter stood motionless in the invisible batter's box as if to say, "Let's do it now." I threw the next couple of pitches back to my brother, who suddenly said, "That's it. None of us feel like playing." I didn't understand what was going on. After all, we had just begun.

My brother dashed over to third base, and from under someone's jacket he pulled out his first Little League trophy. Missing was the gold plate on the front that had identified it. Only the bare marble base remained, and the miniature two-and-a-half-inch high gold-plated baseball player taking his swing. The trophy in its new form was for me.

Summer was ending, and the game was over—forever, as it turned out. Pudge's retirement day had come. The children gathered around and watched my brother give me my prize. I could hardly contain my joy at receiving such a gift. I took the trophy, hopped onto my beloved pink bike, and started down the hill. In his best announcer voice, Joe intoned, "And now, Pudge rides off into her retirement days."

When Carlton Fisk entered the Hall of Fame in the year 2000, he said, "It's not what you achieve in life that defines you, it's what you overcome." Early on, Fisk had a nearly career-ending injury, but he fought his way back to the Big Leagues. I am glad I came to be known as Pudge on our little playground. I think the neighborhood kids wanted to acknowledge in a tangible way what I had overcome when they gave me that trophy. Few experiences in my life are as precious. There is great beauty and wonder in an unexpected and fitting gift. The neighborhood kids and my siblings accepted me, respected me, and faithfully helped me keep on seeing possibilities for new life, and that was their greatest gift of all.

FOUR

The Journey to Self-Acceptance and Self-Love

WE FIND OUR WAY to the mystical vision by taking a healing journey, and ultimately the mystical vision transforms our suffering. Now that we know what it takes to transform our suffering, does our healing journey end?

Let me assure you: the journey is far from over. Once the mystical vision begins to transform our suffering, we are continually challenged to surpass more and more of our brokenness and pain. It's foolish to seek God in our pain in one moment, and then in the next to hate ourselves for not being able to get rid of our brokenness once and for all. But this self-hatred is exactly what can happen if the mystical vision does not penetrate deeply enough into the self to bring acceptance and love.

So where else do we need to travel to make sense of our suffering? Instead of experiencing our transformation as sporadic moments, we seek lasting transformation.

Part of finding God in our pain and suffering is being able to resist the falsehood that our loss is final, and that there are no new opportunities for us to aspire to. As we seek to find God in our pain through inner healing with faithfulness, hope, and love, we have to fight against not only our own inner despair and anguish but also society's negativity. My childhood moments of transformation were largely unhindered by negative influences, but as I grew, I would confront our culture's distorted views about brokenness. To counteract these negative influences, I would have to journey to self-acceptance and even further on to self-love.

Society's negative views toward brokenness unleashed a war against my true self. Slowly but surely, I found myself transfixed by an obsession to unravel all the effects of my disability that made me less likely to fit in. I wanted not so much to be myself but to be normal, to be just like everyone else. Ending the war against ourselves is a struggle for all of us as we face our brokenness. God asks us not only to act in faith in accord with the possibilities in our brokenness but also to accept ourselves unconditionally just as we are. Learning to ignore negative attitudes toward our brokenness will help us find self-acceptance as we keep an opening for transformation alive in our hearts.

Communities can help people accept themselves as they are. I never would have experienced my Wiffle ball retirement day, or the wonder of taking to the streets on my bike, if my siblings and the neighborhood kids had not first accepted me and then supported my efforts at transformation. When a community believes transformation is possible, those with broken bodies find the support they need to surpass their suffering.

But the drama of living in a broken body is played out in a society that expressly devalues brokenness. Our society often determines people's worth by their physical appearance, valuing some body types over others. Overvaluing physical, concrete, observable reality leads to undervaluing inner experience and consciousness, namely, the mystical vision. When society is unable to look beyond what is merely observable, when it is obsessed with beauty and strength, a person with a broken body must struggle uphill. When we, as people with broken bodies, are devalued merely because we cannot meet a superficial cultural ideal, we are challenged to find God and a true sense of self in a deeper and more penetrating reality.

You may be saying to yourself, "But my brokenness is invisible to the world around me." Even if our brokenness is invisible, we still struggle to find true self-acceptance and self-love, because our culture devalues brokenness—all brokenness—so strongly. Whether or not our brokenness is visible to others, our challenge is to turn a blind eye to society's obsession with how we should look or be. Instead, we should look all the more attentively to God for intimacy, help, and guidance. Looking beyond what society says about brokenness, we must seek and find what God would have us know about ourselves. In union with God and deep within ourselves, we will find dignity, beauty, and self-acceptance.

SECOND SURGERY

Tension filled the examining room as my mother and I waited for the doctors to return from their private conference about my future. The doctors had tried to confer quietly, huddled among themselves with us in the room, but we were too curious and apprehensive to ignore them. We heard the word "surgery" several times. The longer the doctors talked, the more difficult it became to contain our questions. As the doctors again pointed to the X-rays, my mother could no longer hold in her curiosity. "Surgery!" she exclaimed. "*What* surgery?"

One of the doctors turned his head away from the pack and said, "Just a minute, Mrs. Ventura." The discussion then shifted from surgery to whether the conversation should be taken outside to the hallway or another examining room.

The doctors took my X-rays and excused themselves, and my mother and I were left alone with our anxiety as the doctors decided my fate. We tried our best to hide from our fear. I colored in my new coloring book, and my mother read a magazine. The minutes seemed like hours as I repeatedly asked to see my mother's watch and annoyed her with questions about when the doctors would return. She tried her best to be patient. "I don't know," she would say. "We will have to wait and see. Use your coloring book." I would stroke the page with my crayons a few times only to find myself staring off aimlessly into space, trying my best to control my anxiety.

Only seven years old, I didn't want more surgery, more pain, more uncertainty. How long would I be sick? I asked myself. Would it hurt as much as last time? Could I possibly be cured this time so I wouldn't have to return to the doctors anymore and I would be well, like all the other children? My mind raced.

After I had asked my mother at least eighteen times when the doctors would return, they waltzed back into the room, my X-rays in hand. "Well, Mrs. Ventura," one of the doctors began, "Diana needs more surgery to lengthen the tendons in her legs so her feet will point outward."

My tears came quickly, and my mother, trying to control her own anxiety, said to me, "Don't you cry." A nurse who had come in with the doctors asked me if she could color with me. I nodded, and she grabbed one of my crayons and joined me. The crayons, the nurse, and my effort to stay within the lines helped me hold back my tears. Soon the tears receded deep inside me, no doubt to visit me on another day. And with my tears now pushed into the depth of my being, I privately resolved to make my disability go away so that I could be normal.

Later in the day, still at Children's Hospital, I fought my anxiety as I was fitted for new night casts. As the warm plaster was being wrapped around my legs, I looked up at the pipes on the basement ceiling and thought, "I am going to beat this. I will show them!" The young doctor making my casts that day was gentle and handsome. As he massaged the plaster into form, I could feel love from the depths of his being seeping into me through his caring hands and kind smile. As the plaster was drying, the nurse from upstairs came down to see how I was doing. She too gave me some peace to help me manage my day.

Getting the casts formed and dried was not nearly as bad as the next step, having them cut in half. The doctor took the buzz saw and began to carve. "Will this be the day they cut through the cast and right through to my leg?" I always thought. My deepest fear in the cast room came when they took the sharp, hooked knife to cut off a window for my toes. I always thought, "Oh, God! This time I'm going to lose my toes for sure." I would peek through a crack in my squinted eyes to be sure my toes were still okay. This time, though, I was not afraid, because I felt love, caring, and gentleness through this doctor's hands. I watched his eyes carefully as he concentrated on his task. I studied his lips and his chin and enjoyed his five o'clock shadow that was much like my father's. I don't know why, at the age of seven, I felt such affection for this man that I remember so vividly years later. Perhaps it is because he, like my Uncle Paul, communicated love and tenderness by doing a simple thing with great care.

Surgery day came after I finished second grade, so it would not disrupt my schooling. I would take the summer to recover and return to school in the fall. This time, I planned to fight. When the doctors put the gas mask over my nose and mouth and told me to count to ten, they were amazed when I actually did. But, alas, I had no choice; the gas was stronger than my will, and off to sleep I went. When I awoke, I could not move my legs. Paralysis is a strange feeling, even if it is due to heavy white plaster. I went back to sleep and slept for a long time. When I awoke, my mother was at my bedside. She was kind and gentle, but I was now determined. Never again would I let anything like this happen to me. Never again would people say to me, "You must go. You must do this or that." I longed for the control to say, "I will not be subjected to anything against my will."

The first night back home from my surgery, I lay in bed wracked with pain. My mother's brother was on his deathbed for the fourth time in a couple years, and my father was engaged in his weekly card game with his buddies downstairs in the kitchen. "Somebody, please help me," I cried out in agony. "Somebody, please! God, I can't believe this."

My cries continued until my father left the game and came up to my bedroom to assess the situation. He stroked my head and said, "What's the matter, baby?"

"Look at my toes," I replied. My big toe was as big as a tangerine. "I am in so much pain, I don't know what to do."

My father said, still stroking my head gently, "Try to relax. Your mother will be home soon."

"Okay," I said. I couldn't remember when I had last taken something for the pain, so I would have to wait for my mother to return and decide when I could have more. My father went back to his buddies, and I managed my pain in a much quieter mode.

The comfort helped a little, because even though it didn't do much for my physical pain, it was nice to have those few stolen moments when I felt less alone in my plight. After a while my mother arrived at my bedside. She, too, for a few moments took the edge off my pain, and then it was off to her duties as the mother of six other children. After that night, I decided there was only one way to escape the pain: holding back all my emotions and feelings, I would fight to make my disability go away and to become normal.

My summer would be anything but normal. My mother and my siblings and I would spend it by my aunt's outdoor, in-ground swimming pool in New Hampshire. Of course I couldn't swim, so all summer I sat and watched as my siblings splashed and played, anticipating the day when I too could swim and play in the water to my heart's content. One day I got so frustrated that I scooted up to the edge of the pool with my casts on, only to be dragged back to my usual spot thirty feet away by my cousin, who laughed and said, "Nice try, Diana. Try again." Exhausted, I sighed and felt private tears hiding behind my eyes. I didn't feel comfortable crying about my disability anymore, so I did not let my tears fall.

Near the end of the summer, the day finally came when my casts were to come off. We drove to Boston and back to New Hampshire the same day and, at about four o'clock on a cloudy, rainy, late August afternoon, I got my wish. Into the pool I went, my legs free of the plaster that had confined them for eight weeks. I ventured out of the shallow end and into the deep, playing with all the imaginary sea monsters, submarines, and pirates that had filled my long afternoons watching from the poolside.

My Aunt Cindy, who had married into the family and originally came from the Deep South, had made her famous Southern fried chicken, and soon everyone else was filling their bellies as I continued to splash in the pool. Finally, seeing that my lips had turned blue and my hands were trembling from the cold, my mother insisted that I get out and partake of some of that scrumptious chicken too. "One, two, three," she said as she swooped me out of the water. My legs were weak from the surgery, and for a moment I stood there trembling. She wrapped me in a towel and quickly picked me up. How beautiful it was, after watching my summer go by, to be allowed, weak legs and all, into the pool to play to my heart's content! And as for the chicken that everyone raved about—it didn't seem nearly as special as swimming in the pool on that late August day.

About eight years later, I walked around that pool with the cousin who had dragged me back from the pool's edge. Forgetting I wasn't normal and couldn't run that fast, I pushed him in, dry clothes and all. I knew that if I could make it into my Aunt Barbara's house and lock myself in her bathroom, I would be safe. I bolted as quickly as I could across her lawn and up a little sandy hill to the door of her side porch. My hand was on the latch when my cousin caught up with me.

I realized what I had done only after he grabbed me. "I'm sorry," I pleaded. "I forgot that I couldn't run! You really don't want to throw me into the pool." My legs and arms flailed, and I screamed as he carried me to the pool like a bride being carried over the threshold. The water wasn't nearly as inviting (nor was it as cold!) as it was on that late August afternoon after my second surgery.

How could I forget that my legs weren't normal and that I couldn't run away? During my childhood (except under special circumstances, such as after my surgery) I was always playing with the neighborhood kids or my siblings, and the other children treated me as normally as possible. It's no surprise to me that I saw myself as normal, even to the point of forgetting that I couldn't run. What do you do when you see someone innocently standing by a pool, fully clothed, on a hot summer afternoon? Especially someone you might secretly resent because years ago, he wouldn't let you join the fun? Of course, you push and run. You just have to realize that if you do that, you are going to get wet!

Thomas Merton writes:

> We speak of "falling in love," as though love were something like water that collects in pools, lakes, rivers, and oceans. You can "fall into" it or walk around it ... You are at a party: you have had more drinks than you need. You decide to walk around the garden a little. You don't notice the swimming pool ... all at once you have to swim! Fortunately, they fish you out, and you are wet but none the worse for wear. Love is like that. If you don't look where you are going, you are liable to land in it: the experience will normally be slightly ridiculous.[1]

I got wet that day when I pushed my cousin into the pool, and love was the reason. True love had made me forget what everyone else would have had me remember of my brokenness and disability. By that time, my inner self had grown so accustomed to who I was that I no longer had to listen to society's telling me I was not normal enough to do what any right-minded fifteen-year-old young woman would do when faced with the opportunity to push and run. If I had listened to all the negative clamoring about the nature and magnitude of my limitations, I would have been doomed from the beginning. Over and over again, people reminded my parents and me that I did not fit society's ideal. "She needs an institution." "She's not smart enough to attend public school." "She won't graduate from high school." "She's not college material." "She won't be able to swim, ride a bike, or ice skate." My ability to ignore and resist this parade of naysayers taught me the essence of self-love.

"Now don't get your hopes up too high," we have all heard. But what's the difference between believing unrealistically high expectations and believing the myriad negative predictions thrown at us from every side? The truth is that no one has the right to say what we can and cannot do. No one knows what the outcome may be. Sure, there are many things I will never be able to do. Perhaps I will never make it to the top of Everest, but that is for me to discover and work out with God. How will I muster up the confidence to do what I am truly capable of doing if I listen to the negative voices all around me, telling me what I can't do?

In whatever I undertake, whether to climb Everest or to walk around my block, I must muster up the courage and confidence to try. The same holds true for you. The only way to discover your abilities is to try, and because others may not see your life and circumstances as you do, you

---

1. Thomas Merton, *Love and Living*, ed. Naomi Burton Stone and Patrick Hart (San Diego: Harcourt, Brace, Jovanovich, 1985) 25.

must be willing to ignore their negative predictions. As you close off the negative voices, you will be free to pursue faithfully the things that God has given you to do. As we walk with God, seeking to meet the challenges our brokenness gives us, we must also enter into a deeper and more lasting relationship with ourselves. For as society rejects us, we must fight all the more to find our way to self-acceptance and self-love.

FIRST GRADE

I filed into the classroom like all the other first-graders even though I was still officially in kindergarten. I took a seat on the edge of my brother Paul's chair as he sat with his legs open so I would have a place to sit. "Do you have enough room?" he asked.

"Yup," I replied confidently. He held me affectionately around my waist as he smiled at his teacher. He was proud to have his little sister with him. As a child, Paul was mischievous, but he also had a strong loving streak. The two traits often played against each other. One spring day when he was a small boy, he picked all of our next-door neighbor's tulips, then rang her doorbell and gave them to her as a bouquet. Mrs. Clancy, God bless her soul, took the flowers with joy and didn't reprimand him. My mother later, and rather forcefully, explained to Mrs. Clancy that Paul (even though he gave the flowers to her with a sweet smile) probably knew full well what he was doing. He must have realized that the only way out of the mess he had gotten himself into by picking the tulips was to ring the doorbell and smile for all he was worth. Perched on the edge of his seat, I was lucky to find myself on his loving side.

The teacher, Mrs. Jane, asked a question. I knew the answer and my hand shot up, but she did not call on me. Continually throughout the morning she ignored my raised hand. My fate was already sealed. I would go to the Industrial School for Crippled Children because school officials had convinced my parents that it would be better for me to be with those who could truly help me. After all, I was not performing up to par.

I had no idea that I would not attend elementary school with my brothers and sisters. In 1970, disabled children did not attend regular public schools. My parents tried to get school officials to let me into the public school that was just a mile from our house, but the officials had other plans. They did not want to deal with me, and they would be sure to make their plans work out, regardless of my intelligence.

At the Industrial School for Crippled Children, most of the children were defined as "less than"—less-than-healthy physical bodies, less-than-intelligent minds, less than everything. The school administrators believed they were doing students a favor by teaching them a trade; after all, these disabled children were not college material. Teachers had preconceived notions of what the children could or could not do, and so they defined their futures for them. Just as white culture tried to define black people as "nobodies," these educators tried to define people with disabilities as people of little worth.

The black community found its identity through the Black Power movement and the Civil Rights Movement, and these movements laid the groundwork for those of us with disabilities to find our identity too. The *Brown v. Board of Education* ruling and other civil rights work helped bring to fruition Chapter 766, a Massachusetts law guaranteeing free appropriate education for disabled children. Enacted in 1972, the law opened the door for me to be mainstreamed into public schools. Shortly after Chapter 766 was passed, a federal law (PL 94–142) following the same guidelines allowed children all over the country to attend public school. The Civil Rights Movement is one of the most important reasons why I can write this book today. On the backs of all those who marched, I found my opportunity for freedom.

James Cone, author of *Black Theology and Black Power*, describes white racists' misunderstanding of black people as "*existential absurdity*."[2] Existential absurdity arises when black people meet a white world that prefers to define black people as things rather than as people. Existential absurdity arose in me when school officials, with no basis for doing so, sent me off to the special school where I would be defined as less capable than "normal" people. But people with disabilities, like black people, do not see or believe themselves to be less than everyone else. I knew the answers to the teacher's questions on the day I visited my brother's first-grade classroom; no one can ever take that away from me. The school officials could not have been more wrong about my learning ability. I now exceed many of them in earned degrees and, more important, in wisdom.

To make matters worse, school officials continued to make mistaken predictions: "She's not really college material. She really should go to vocational high school." Wrong, wrong, wrong . . . and absurd. I am here to

2. James H. Cone, *Black Theology and Black Power* (Maryknoll, NY: Orbis, 1997) 11 (italics added).

tell you loud and clear—don't believe all those negative predictions; they simply aren't true. People prefer to believe what makes them comfortable, not what allows them—or others—to stretch.

When confronted with a society that wishes to define you or a part of you in a false way, it is time to resist. The civil rights movement began with an act of resistance on December 1, 1955, when Rosa Parks, an unknown seamstress from Montgomery, Alabama, refused to budge from her bus seat so that a white person could sit down. Accused of violating a city ordinance, she was arrested and fined.

Rosa Parks was able to resist because she knew and believed in her own truth. She knew she had a right to sit at the front of the bus, so she did not act on the lie society told her about herself, the lie that because of her black skin, she had less worth than white people. For me, the lie was that because of my physical disability, I was unable to keep up intellectually with able-bodied children. Her act of resistance helped spark the Civil Rights Movement that would change my life.

My mother taught me to resist anyone who tried to label me. She taught me to question unequivocally any negative predictions about my life. She refused to believe that my cerebral palsy would diminish who I would become. She never dimmed the light of my dreams by saying, "You will never . . ." Instead, she encouraged me to dream big. The sky was the limit. "You'll be a long-distance runner one day; you'll see," she would say. When people stared at me, she allowed me to confront them. I was privy more than once to her angry confrontations of any doctors who, in their presumption of superiority, thought little of me. My mother simply did not tolerate anyone who entertained ideas of my being "less than" everyone else because of my cerebral palsy, so later in life I refused to tolerate such ideas as well.

From my mother I learned what to resist; from God, I received the power to resist. God teaches us to resist society's falsehoods and reveals to us our true identity. Only a person who knows she is beloved by God can resist lies such as "She won't amount to anything—throw her into an institution."

It is unfortunate that my parents did not initially resist the school officials when I was to enter first grade. I once asked my mother why she let such a thing happen to me. She explained, "I am sorry. Everyone convinced me it was what would be best for you. I didn't know it was going to set you back." But set me back it did! At the Industrial School for Crippled

Children, I learned very little, and when I entered a regular classroom two years later, everyone's prediction came true. My misperceived ability became a self-fulfilling prophecy, and I lagged behind my classmates academically. School officials were unable to see my potential until the law mandated them to do so. And even then, school would be a struggle until I reached college and found teachers who truly believed in and nurtured my intellect. I earned my first degree and marched on to get a few more. But it was the law that first opened up the door to my education and truly saved my life. May I always remember that my life today is thanks to every person who fought for civil rights.

Civil rights seek to give everyone a fair shake regardless of individual differences. People with physical disabilities and brokenness are excluded from opportunities offered to others in society and some of this stems from people misconstruing the meaning of physical disabilities and brokenness.

Society around us was saying, "No, Mrs. Ventura, your daughter will never amount to anything. No, Mrs. Ventura, your daughter won't be able to learn. No, Mrs. Ventura, your daughter will never move very well. No, Mrs. Ventura, your daughter will never ride a bike. No, Mrs. Ventura, your daughter will never ice skate. No, Mrs. Ventura, your daughter will not enjoy life playing with the other neighborhood kids." My mother would have none of it; she acted faithfully on her commitment to me as she sought to give me as normal a childhood as possible. In doing so, my mother said yes to all the possibilities life could offer me, unknowingly paving the way for miracles.

Society misunderstands brokenness; more often than not, people see what is lost in brokenness rather than God's ability to work in it; diminished value rather than opportunities for love. Thomas Merton warns that our notions of love are affected by media images. Without realizing it, we have what he calls "a package concept of love" in which "love is regarded as a deal":

> In order to make a deal you have to appear in the market with a worthwhile product, or if the product is worthless, you can get by if you dress it up in a good-looking package. We unconsciously think of ourselves as objects for sale on the market. We want to be wanted.... Hence, we waste a great deal of time modeling ourselves on the images presented to us by an affluent marketing society.[3]

3. Merton, *Love and Living*, 28–29.

In our market-driven-love economy, the question becomes, how well does your body fit society's idealized package? The drive to have a perfect body (i.e., a perfect package) urges people to tummy tucks, breast implants, facelifts, and nose jobs. People want to improve their package so they can raise their value and increase their opportunities for love exchanges. Brokenness diminishes the value of the package and thereby also diminishes the person's potential for love. In this deal-making economy, people with thoughts, feelings, and souls become objectified—that is, they are treated as mere things. Their value is seen as directly proportional to their ability to conform to the idealized image. The trouble is, of course, that bodily appearance is not a reliable means of evaluating a person's capacity to give and receive love.

By *love* I am not speaking exclusively about the sensual love of *eros*, but also about the companionable love of *philia*, the affectionate love of *storgē*, and the unconditional love of *agapē*. (The Greeks wisely used multiple words for this many-splendored phenomenon.) Opportunities for friendship are a part of being accepted in our communities as persons with dignity and worth. When society limits our value and denies us love, it becomes hard for us to sustain a sense of self-worth and self-acceptance.

When I was young, I knew a girl I will call Lisa. Lisa was born with a growth protruding out of her right eye socket, leaving a tiny slit showing only the white part of her eye. Lisa is not physically beautiful, and so society questions her dignity and worth. When she goes out in public, she encounters people who shrink back in horror. Every day Lisa struggles to be known as a complete and whole human being. Joseph Merrick, the "Elephant Man," had the same problem. When a crowd of people pulled his mask off, he had to remind them that he was not a monster by screaming, "I am a human being!" Our society sees little value in relating to people like Lisa and Merrick, because they do not fit our idealized image of what gives a person worth. If Joseph Merrick were with us today, would we saw and tuck his head, straighten his back, and alter his face until it looked normal? By looking like everyone else, would he find his place in society, his value restored? But after his body was all tucked and clipped, who would Joseph Merrick be?

Theologian David Tracy writes, "The final indignity for anyone is to be forbidden of one's own voice or to be robbed of one's own experience."[4] I had the opportunity to ask him about this sentence, and he kindly elaborated: "I was walking home one day when I saw a man picking through the trash. I felt that it was my duty to help the poor man. I reached in my wallet and pulled out a ten-dollar bill. When I tried to give it to the man he said to me, 'I don't need your money. Who are you to give me ten dollars? I am just fine the way I am.'"[5] Tracy walked away perplexed, pondering the meaning of the man's refusal. As I was growing up, I engaged in a constant battle to preserve and assert my dignity. More than anything, I wanted to be normal, to walk just like everyone else, and to be accorded the same dignity and respect as any other human being—as someone who is broken and yet whole. When others looked at me, I wanted them to see and know me just as they saw and knew everyone else. I wanted to be loved, not for conforming to society's expectations, but for who I was.

IS IT A SHAME?

One day I was walking down a busy street, wearing nice clothes and with my hair all done up, and I passed a bearded man. When he looked at me, he wagged his head and said, "It's a shame!"

His words stopped me in my tracks. I thought, "That was really rude." I knew exactly what he was referring to—the very noticeable sway in my gait. My next thought came in a split second: "Do I want to do anything about it?" My answer was an emphatic yes, so I turned around and ran after him as fast as I could.

It was an effort to catch up with him, because he was moving quickly. Nearly out of breath, I called out, "Hey, Buddy, *you're* a shame. I'm more beautiful than the bigotry in your heart will ever see." The man did not respond.

I turned and walked away silently and slowly, trying to regain my composure and put myself back together, wishing upon this man anything that would teach him to overcome his bigotry. I was glad I had confronted him; but wow, I had to think as I walked away, is it a shame? Am I a shame?

4. David Tracy, *Plurality and Ambiguity: Hermeneutics, Religion, Hope* (San Francisco: Harper & Row, 1987) 103.

5. Personal communication with David Tracy, 2002.

It's amazing how quickly a complete stranger could cast a shadow of self-doubt over me, even after I had vehemently stood up to him. This is how existential absurdity seeps into the soul. Only the street-savvy emerge unharmed from the constant negative onslaught. Such encounters are injected into everyday experience with such subtlety that we hardly realize what's happening until it's over. My mind continued to wrestle with the man's words: "I mean, I know I am not a shame, but is it a shame that I walk this way? Would I be more beautiful if I were normal?"

The tactless bearded man was merely reflecting the way our society thinks, proving the validity of Merton's observations about our package concept of love. Many people would see me as more lovable if my body conformed to the standard of normality that most bodies adhere to. Longing to be valuable in the love marketplace, I felt a constant desire to be as normal as possible.

How hard it is to think of ourselves as beautiful when people around us wag their heads as if we are a shame. Most of us cannot get the medical makeover that would make us "normal," and in any case, why does our culture think beauty means obliterating all forms of physical difference? It seems to me that as people work their way through the assembly line of plastic surgery, they forget that love is more than a deal to be made.

Beauty is what gives pleasure through the senses, especially through sight. When we seek to make ourselves beautiful only on the outside, we forget the true worth of what makes us beautiful on the inside. Now, don't get me wrong; there is a real distinction between the beautiful and the ugly. I am not saying, "We are all beautiful on the inside," as if to say to those who make little effort to care for themselves, "You are beautiful, too." Some people are *not* beautiful on the inside, and some think too little care of themselves to make their outer appearance as pleasing as possible.

However, those who strive to be who they are before God are beautiful, regardless of their bodily condition. Joseph Merrick's distorted and deformed body was not beautiful, but Joseph Merrick the man shows us something about real, lasting beauty. Was this man capable of love in spite of his loss? "I am a human being," he said. Regardless of his broken body, Merrick was no different from the rest of us. We all need to be loved, treated with dignity, and seen as beautiful. What made him a man of outstanding beauty was his courage to carry himself with dignity, knowing he had the right to be loved and treated as a whole human being despite society's fear and disgust. When we have the courage to see beyond the deal-making, package concept of love, we discover the true meaning of beauty.

How should we characterize beauty if we are not to define it in physical terms? One aspect of beauty to consider is how well a person or thing conforms to its own nature. How well did Carlo Carretto, Jacques Lusseyran, or Edith Barfoot conform to the persons God called them to be? How well do I conform to the Diana God wants me to be? Are you being all the person God asks you to be?

It is easy to want to change all kinds of things about ourselves. We think that if we do this or that, or if God would just answer our prayer for healing, we will be new and improved, special, even beautiful. But is that new and improved person the one God is calling us to be?

It can be hard to discern who we are truly meant to be. I think the secret is hidden somewhere in the depths of our limitations. If we push ourselves to our limits in the name of God, then where we end up is where we are meant to be. If you study as hard as you can, and all you come up with are Bs, then you are meant to be a B student. It is difficult to be in the middle or at the end of the pack when all we want to do is win, but God calls us to accept who we are with joy. If we are willing, God will lead us to self-acceptance.

Longing to be normal, I needed God to lead me to self-acceptance.

PASSIONATE KISSES

When I was a teenager, I wanted more than anything in the world to have the same romances as my peers. In the eighth grade, there was a boy—I'll call him Joe B.—whom all the girls had a crush on, and of course I had one too. He sat in the back of our science class. Many of the girls found any excuse they could to spin around on their lab stools to stare at him.

Mr. Burnham, our science teacher (complete with horn-rimmed eyeglasses and white plastic pocket protector), knew full well of Joe B.'s popularity, so he often called on Joe B. to volunteer for experiments: that way, he would be sure to get our attention. When I turned around to watch those experiments, I was looking straight at three of the most popular girls with their perfect hair, bodies, and clothes. These girls used every opportunity to make fun of me. Mostly, they would whisper little jabs about the way I looked. When I would spin around to confront them, they would stop their childish whispering. In their minds, not only were they better than me, they were superior to everyone else.

One of these girls would soon date Joe B. Of course he would never date me, not with my twisted and deformed body. And I knew it too. As we watched this handsome man in the making take part in all those experiments, pouring this and stirring that, all of us in the class knew our place in society.

Several years later, when I was nineteen, my siblings and I gave a party to celebrate the coming of the New Year. A mournful haze hung over our celebration, because it was the first year since my father had died suddenly, at the young age of fifty, of a massive heart attack. Now we were forced to live without the playful and loving man who had influenced us all so greatly. My father was a determined man. He dreamed big, learned from his mistakes, and worked hard for what he wanted. He loved his family with disciplined care and even reverence, and he worked many long hours so he could amply provide for all his children. We were never in want of anything essential.

Having grown up in poverty, my father became a millionaire as a self-employed builder and developer, but he maintained a humble spirit. He wore a worn-out, old, heavy green coat during the winter months that made him look like a bum. At his building site, he'd be right in there getting dirty with the rest of his workers. No sense in being pretentious about being the developer of the building project—he felt he wasn't any more important than the guy working next to him. He simply wanted to make his dreams come true, and his biggest dreams were always for his family.

So my father's spirit hung around with us as we tried to be as joyful as he would have wanted us to be, even though our hearts were aching at the memory of his playful antics that had filled our household. All the teasing and tickling were ended; we'd have no more mischievous pokes and giggles. My siblings and I would have to reach beyond our sadness and grief on that first New Year's Eve without him and still have a little fun. I think we all just pretended we still loved life, or perhaps we did not know yet how deep the rivers of grief so painfully run.

One of the invited guests was Joe B. I tried not to pay obsessive attention to him, although I couldn't help remembering science class. And, yes, I noticed, he did grow up to be as handsome as I had imagined he would. As midnight and the coming New Year grew closer, the champagne flowed, and we all became increasingly cheerful. Many of us gathered by the TV in the den to watch the ball drop in Times' Square. My siblings and the other guests were in pairs, except for Joe B. and, of course, me, as

we counted down: ten, nine, eight, seven, six, five, four, three, two, one—
Happy New Year!

As the ball dropped, everyone kissed their partner. I stood in the
middle of the den wondering, "Now what am I supposed to do?" The kiss-
ing seemed to go on for an eternity. Suddenly, someone called my name.
As I spun around to see who it could be, a strong arm took me by the
waist, and handsome Joe B.'s lips found mine.

When our long, passionate kiss ended, the room was spinning. I don't
know whether it was from the kiss or the champagne—probably a little of
both. I really was off balance. I staggered away, swaying even more deeply
than usual from the wonder of that ardent kiss. We both knew it was only
a kiss. Afterward, he went his way, and I went mine. But I couldn't help
wondering what those "perfect" girls in science class would think if they
could see me now, for I was the one who got his New Year's Eve kiss for
1984. I went to bed shortly after midnight, dreaming of the day my true
love would find me, to hold me and kiss me all the night through.

On that night, a few crumbs of physical intimacy fell from my master's
table. And yet what should a starving person do? When the crumbs fall,
you eat. Throughout my life, opportunities for physical intimacy would
come few and far between. A few other passionate kisses have come my
way, and I have treasured the physical closeness of those moments.

In light of Merton's package concept of love, I am damaged goods.
Who wants to buy something if the container is torn or dented? Perhaps
if I looked normal, Joe B. would have dated me. Maybe to him and to the
rest of the world, I am not beautiful enough as I am. With my disabled legs
moving this way and that, I may be seen as someone to admire or even to
be inspired by, but not to passionately love. No, no, no, Joe B. could not see
me as someone to date. How would he have contended with the ridicule?
"Hey, couldn't you get a normal girl?" some of the other kids would have
said. Dating me requires sacrifice. Truth is, who wants to contend with
the fact that I can't go mountain biking or take to the slopes in Aspen? So
I certainly understand why I never found myself in Joe B.'s arms late into
the night.

Often our brokenness leaves us feeling rejected and unloved. We
want with our whole heart and being to know ourselves as beautiful and
as capable of love, and yet many of us are alone. We feel that some aspect
of our brokenness is standing in the way of intimacy, and we long for it to
be removed. "If God would only fix this part of me, I know I would find

the love I need," we say to ourselves. Our complaints go on and on as we seek a remedy for our painful loneliness.

And even if we do find ourselves in the arms of a loved one, it always seems as if our brokenness somehow interferes with the deeper sense of love we long to feel. Again we think, "If that pesky bit of brokenness could be removed and put out of my way forever, I would experience the fullness of love that I long for." On and on it goes. It doesn't matter who we are—normal or disabled, thin or obese, tall or short, or whatever. If we're human, we are broken, and we're all seeking to get rid of the brokenness that we think denies us the love we want and deserve.

Truly, all this fighting against our brokenness breeds in us a strong sense of self-hatred.

Society hates brokenness, weakness, and the fragility of the human condition. Perhaps I blame society for my loneliness when the fault is actually my own. Perhaps I have absorbed society's contempt and have turned it against myself. The feeling, whether true or not, remains: any form of brokenness, weakness, or imperfection may leave me in a world without love. At times my heart is heavy with loneliness. Too many hopes have been dashed upon the rocks of despair; too many precious dreams casually tossed into oblivion.

When our brokenness leaves us without someone to be close to, loneliness closes in on us. Fear, anger, and rage are likely to follow us around. We hate ourselves for what we cannot change. To end this cycle of self-hatred, we must find our way to self-acceptance by embracing our brokenness. As we begin our healing journey, our mystical vision and growing intimacy with God open up the way for this embrace. When we act faithfully, as God would wish, to make the most of ourselves within the confines of our brokenness, peace over our brokenness seeps into our souls as inner healing begins to take hold.

At the age of nineteen when I kissed Joe B., I longed to be normal. I was still fighting with all my might against my brokenness. But God would teach me that the answer is not found in fighting or removing our brokenness, but rather in embracing and making peace with it.

BASKETBALL

When I was fourteen, I began a physical training program to make myself as normal as possible. The doctor at Children's had proposed another surgery that didn't seem right to me. The surgery would entail moving a muscle from one part of my leg to another. I was overweight and out of shape, and in the car on the way home from the appointment, I said to my mother, "This doesn't sound right. I'm going to get in shape, and then let's see if I need surgery."

I began walking around my dead-end street, up the hills and around the circle. Four laps equaled a mile. They were hilly miles, four hills per lap, plus the circle. When you're a kid, you don't care, and I didn't. I was back in my "mountain-moving" mode of walking in faith with God. This time, I intuitively knew I could not fail.

My days soon were packed with endless training sessions. Weight-lifting, biking, calisthenics, walking, running, and swimming were all part of my regular workout routine. I would like to say that getting out of the surgery was my primary motive, but it wasn't. Truth is, I was in love—in love with basketball. My constant ambition was to play on the girls' basketball team at my high school, Northeast Metropolitan Regional Vocational School.

I had been sent to vocational school under the supposition that I was not college material. This turned out to be untrue, but attending Northeast gave me the opportunity to play sports. Northeast enrolled substantially fewer girls than boys, so none of the girls' teams had cuts to make the squad. All I had to do was try to make myself as good a player as possible, and I would be in. I might not play very much, but I would make the team.

Soon the summer days grew shorter, and I returned to Northeast as a thinner and much more agile sophomore. I had dropped twenty-five pounds, no small feat for someone who is barely five feet tall. I was ready to integrate school into my training regime, but my true goal was to play basketball and play it well. I spent my weekends, afternoons, and nights playing basketball at our backyard net. When the light of day wore thin, I'd simply turn on our floodlights to continue my practice. If I didn't make all my foul shots, I made myself run more laps around the street. Tirelessly I worked. Finally, right after Thanksgiving, our practices were to begin.

Basketball players do all kinds of things to get ready for their games. One drill is running wind sprints. Everyone lines up along the baseline of one of the baskets. When the coach blows the whistle, you have to sprint as fast as you can to the foul line, or what would be the foul line if you were not lined up right under the basket when you started. Once you touch the foul line, you have to sprint back to the baseline, where you started, and then touch that line. Then you need to sprint again to half court, touch the line, and run all the way back again to the baseline. Once at the baseline, you have to keep running as fast as you can back to the foul line on the other side of the court, and then back to the original baseline, and then back again and, yes, one more time up the court, to touch the baseline on the other side of the court, and then back again.

The coach of the Northeast Knights girls' basketball team, Mrs. Christine Dodge, blew the whistle and away we went. "Wow, I am way behind," I thought, as I still was at half court coming back when the other girls were running for the foul line farthest from us. "I've got to catch up," I thought, as I was one full court-length behind when the next-slowest girl finished her sprint. I came in last, even after all the training.

Rude awakening! Nothing had prepared me for the fact that once I set foot on the basketball court, I would be truly "disabled" again. I had become so accustomed to my disability's making no difference—at least in my daily functioning, because in my everyday life I could keep up with everyone else—that I was shocked to find my deficits still looming so large.

I realized then that I was not who I wanted to be. I wanted to be normal, to run and play basketball like all the other players. Just as I had wanted to be like my siblings, I now wanted to be like my comrades on the basketball team. The people changed, but the dream remained the same: to be normal. That was my heart's longing. It's not that I wanted God to swoop down with a magic wand and make it all better. I was willing to put my time in. The miles I ran and the time I spent obsessively exercising were meant to say to God, "I am willing to work to move this mountain, piece by piece."

All this mountain-moving activity awakened my love for God. I think that when you are willing to work through life's challenges, God meets you with grace and intimacy. After my training sessions, I would sit on the retaining wall next to our driveway up a ways from the basketball net. There, under a young maple tree, I would lie back and dreamily look at the sky through the leaves, or I would sit upright staring off into the distance at the streetlights and the hill and the circle. In those times of reflection, I often found myself praying to God.

As a youngster, I had prayed with fervor for the effects of my broken-ness and disability to be undone. But as I prayed, I sensed that God was not magically going to make me normal one day. Now that I was older, I was discovering another form of prayer. I talked with God as if the Divine One were my best friend sitting next to me; and a sense of intimacy, a bond of trust, grew within me. I felt God's love touching every part of my experience. During my runs and exercises, and again on that sacred patch of land around our backyard basketball net, God was with me. I could feel God's presence in my movement, in my muscles in spasm from too much exertion, in my new and improved running times, and in the shot missed so many times but now made. My dream, basketball, and God were one. And that is why I can say I was in love.

It was not a silly exaggeration; not even childhood naiveté. Instead, it was miracle making in action. As my body grew stronger, my heart discovered a deeper and more urgent longing for God. Basketball and the drive to overcome my disability were pushing me closer to God. Love flowed from my every spin: from my tiny jump shots when my feet barely left the ground, to my long hook shot and the endless sweat pouring from my brow.

Awaken, you muscles, so silent and asleep. Awaken, I tell you! For I am traveling. I have a dream. I have places to go, and you, my broken body, are coming with me. Out from your slumber now, all your movements so sacred and holy that I imagine in my dreams. Come to life now. I demand it! God is with me. Emerge, emerge, I am willing to work. I am willing to do hard things—I am willing to run extra. I am willing to pound out that extra set of exercises. Work with me now, all you muscles, my body says. Yes, I am talking to you about all those things you've longed to do. Come out, come out, you can do it. Work hard and try.

These were my thoughts all those years ago.

I have to tell the truth, though: my disability taught me to respect my limits. Many days, my limits were all I experienced. Ah, but this is how sacred this time was for me—because God was with me so much, I could enjoy the journey anyway. I loved the fight, so I fought. And yes, frustration followed me around, and rage came easily when my limitations blocked my wishes. But with God at my side, a sense of awe and wonderment stayed with me, whatever I was trying to achieve. I had long since averted the proposed surgery, and this of course pleased my mother. Now I focused my attention completely on trying to undo as much of my disability as I could. And in the meantime, I played some basketball.

On the day of our first game, I sat on the bench for nearly the entire time. I came home for dinner, and as we always did, the eight of us and my parents sat down for our meal together. Then the questions began: How was your game? Did you play? Did you score any points?

I jumped from my seat, swearing. "I can't take life in this f***ing body anymore! Why did God make me this way anyway? Doesn't anybody care about how hard I f***ing try?"

The family followed me into the living room through a large open doorway that led from our dining area. My father faced me, his hand raised. I thought he was going to strike me, but instead he put his hand firmly on my shoulder and looked into my tear-filled eyes. "Can we talk about this?" he asked.

After I told what had happened—that I had sat on the bench nearly the whole time and had played for barely one second—the rest of the family returned to their meal. My father stayed with me. He said something similar to Carlton Fisk: "It's not what you achieve in life that defines you, it's what you overcome." I far surpassed everyone else on both teams, my father explained, because of what I had overcome.

I went scoreless my first season. For the most part, I just sat and watched the other girls play. What I wanted for myself continued to wreak havoc within me. I could not understand why my dreams weren't coming true after I had I put so much time into them. I was frustrated that my life was not conforming to my every desire. Why wasn't I getting more playing time? "After all that work," I would say to myself. "After all that work."

I had tried to keep myself focused on the wonder of the journey, and when I did, I found God. But every time my focus shifted from the joy of the journey to the pain of my own unfulfilled wants and desires, I lost my sense of inner balance and of God. I lost my appreciation of my awakening body with its new ways to move. I could now get up from sitting on the floor by pushing off the floor with my hand as if I were going into a backbend, and up I'd go on two sturdy legs as if I were normal. (I can still see myself getting up that way, though now that I am not in such great shape, I have to turn around on all fours, put myself in linebacker position, and push off with the hand that's on the ground.) When I was young, I had no idea how amazing all of these new movements were. The more I was led by my own agenda for my accomplishments, the more anger, rage, and frustration filled me.

The entire summer, I trained with fanatical fervor. My activity was nearly constant. Morning, noon, and night the beat went on. I ran wind sprints up the hills on our dead end-street, nearly twenty-five miles a week. I biked another ten miles and swam at least two. I taught myself to jump rope so that I could do three revolutions. I could jump nearly six inches into the air, and I could bang out fifty of the most perfect pushups anyone has ever seen. To my broken body, it was as if I had made the Olympic team.

There were moments in my basketball career that gave me that same Olympic feeling. Believe it or not, one such moment came during a practice. As I returned for my junior year and my second season, I had no idea how my efforts to improve my performance were going to pan out. During my prayers before the season, a feeling of deeper and more lasting self-acceptance had come over me. I knew what God was asking me to do: relax, try hard, and have fun. Could I do that? Would it affect my game?

Coach blew the whistle and, like horses in a race, we were off: "Wow, I touched the foul line and then the baseline! I'm keeping up, all right. We're at half-court now, and I'm not lagging behind. Okay, back to the original baseline. Wow, I might make it, just two full lengths of the court to go. Got to get to the baseline at the far end of the court. Here we come. There are people behind me, and—yes—Diana crosses the finish line with four girls behind her! Four girls in an all-out footrace! *I won, I won, I won!*"

I couldn't believe that had just happened, and I didn't even care when Coach said, "You girls have to pick up the pace. You're really slow. Diana beat a couple of you." I had reached the mark. For one split second of my life, I was normal and I knew it. I savored the taste as we all stood at the baseline, huffing and puffing, awaiting our coach's further instructions. She said, "You all run it again, only quicker. Diana, you go outside in the hall and take a moment. That was absolutely amazing."

It *was* amazing, I know, because it never happened again.

The difference between where I started and where I ended up was truly remarkable. No one would have dreamed it when I was lying in my cast, but here it had become my reality. God and I had collaborated to make it so. I went out into the hallway and prayed to God in thanksgiving. I looked through the large plate-glass windows at the courtyard, the sun, the grass, the sky, the clouds. Everything felt sacred, just as it had that day long ago on the swing. I knew this feeling would last but a moment, but ah, what a beautiful moment to remember for a lifetime!

How wonderful to be sent out into the hallway to ponder what had just happened, to solidify the moment in my consciousness, allowing it to have a lasting impact. My momentary normality came to me as a gift from God. Being willing to work within my situation had moved a mountain. Yes, it was not quite the way I had wanted it to be. We like to imagine exaggerated triumphs, like my coming in first with everyone else behind me always and forever, never to lose again. Instead, my triumph gave me one beautiful moment to last a lifetime. Would it be such a beautiful moment with such lasting meaning if I were normal? There are benefits to being just who we are.

Through all the rest of the practices, the girls continued to beat me, but I made remarkable progress. I lagged only a few steps behind. Longing to avenge my scoreless season of the previous year, I had again worked tirelessly throughout the summer and early fall. Our first game of the 1981–1982 season came at a small Catholic high school, Presentation of Mary Academy. We were playing in the lowest division, where little basketball programs played other small programs. Beyond that, I was on the junior-varsity team. The stakes were much simpler in these down-home games, and that's one reason I got to play. We filed into the gym, and I noticed a crucifix hanging on the wall. I took it as a good sign that I might actually meet my goal of scoring. I prayed as I did when I was learning to ride a bike, "Please, God, let this be the day."

Coach signaled for me to go into the game at the beginning of the second quarter. I went out onto the court, playing shooting guard. Our team brought the ball up. I moved to get the ball and had a wide-open shot. Two dribbles and up I went with my new and improved jump shot where my feet could really leave the ground. As the ball rattled through the basket, the entire gym erupted with cheers. Coach was still not confident in my ability to play, however. I didn't score any more during that game, because she quickly took me out.

After the game, two heavyset nuns hurled themselves from the stands and rushed toward me, their white habits flying in the air behind them like capes. They encircled me with an intense embrace, squeezing me tightly between them, drowning my face in their breasts. As the teams cleared out, we huddled in the middle of the gym to pray. My head settled onto the chest of one of the nuns as if it were a shelf. The other nun stood close to us. The nun on whose chest my head was lying did most of the praying. Holding my head gently to her bosom, she began to cry out for God's holiness to come and visit us. As the prayers took form and shape on her lips, she would let my head up for a second from time to time to look into my eyes. She then would rest my head back down onto her chest. The prayers went something like this: "God, you have blessed this child. God, continue to bless this child. Keep her safe, holy, and healthy . . ." As these two nuns prayed over me, I felt the holiness of God touch me through their love. I am sure that the blessings from their prayers still abound.

ACCEPTANCE AND AUTHENTICITY

As my basketball career was drawing to a close during my senior year, I had yet to find true and full self-acceptance. I still wanted more than anything to be normal, to be ordinary, to be like everyone else. I just wanted all my limitations to go away. Yet when we continue to fight our brokenness, we actually turn away from ourselves. We believe that our brokenness robs us of our true selves. We don't fit with the package that sells in the love market, and so we believe ourselves to be damaged, defective, worthless goods. Quite the opposite is actually true.

While all this fighting within myself was going on, God sought to teach me something different through moments of beauty: my passionate kiss, my winning the all-out footrace, the triumph of my scoring. Even though these moments were not entirely what I would have wished for, they were the moments I had. Whenever we see glimmers of beauty, self-acceptance moves closer to us. It's as if these moments say to us, "Here I am! Look at me. Acknowledge me." As we reflect on our beautiful moments, we find even more beauty lingering in our brokenness. And when we are able to see beauty in our own lives, we begin to understand the true love-making qualities of our Creator. God dispels our self-hatred by illuminating the beauty hiding in our brokenness. Self-acceptance begins to take hold as we let these moments of beauty inform our souls, and we find ourselves engaged in a sacred embrace with God.

Once we catch a glimpse of the beauty hiding in our brokenness, we are able to look beyond the deal-making concept of love perpetuated by society. Our culture does not make it easy to see the beauty in brokenness, because it always wants things to fit into its own preconceived ideas of what is good and real. And what is good, according to our culture? How about a perfect body, one with not even a lingering trace of human frailty? Thomas Merton believed that true love does away with deal-making, with striving to be perfect so that we can be worthy of love: "My true meaning and worth are shown to me not in my estimate of myself, but in the eyes of the one who loves me; and that one must love me as I am, with my faults and limitations, revealing to me the truth that these faults and limitations cannot destroy my worth in *their* eyes; and that I am therefore valuable as a person, in spite of my shortcomings, in spite of the imperfections of my exterior 'package.'"[6]

Some people looking out onto the basketball court at Presentation of Mary Academy saw a poor disabled young woman trying to play, but the nuns who prayed over me so fervently saw me differently. They saw with spiritual eyes, and their mystical vision revealed the truth. When I was seventeen, I failed to realize that if my legs moved just like everyone else's, I wouldn't have received such beautiful blessings upon my scoring success. The precious moments that my broken body had given me would have been wiped away in an instant, along with all their sacred lessons.

Instead of tragedy, my broken body gives me moments of beauty that I can ponder for a lifetime. And in my heart of hearts I know that God would not want the wonder of my small but meaningful triumphs, like winning the footrace, obliterated in the name of normality. Instead, through me, and according to my true nature, God wishes to reveal something of the meaning of beauty. My body, just by being broken and disabled, speaks of the beauty of our individual uniqueness.

Our brokenness gives us something that the others do not have: a full and complete grasp on reality. Brokenness teaches us the truth by keeping our feet planted firmly on the ground. It releases us from the lie that our culture would have us believe: that we can—and should—be invincible, unstoppable, completely and unquestionably perfect and sound in every respect. Every day as I teeter and sometimes fall, I am reminded of just how frail the human condition is. Truly, people struggling with brokenness are the first to say, "The emperor has no clothes."

When our brokenness exposes the truth that we are not invincible, we are free to embrace the truth of our weakness, failings, and shortcomings. We no longer have to believe society's lie that in order to be worthy of love, we must have perfect bodies and minds and never show any flaws or admit to any limitations. Leaving behind the falsehood, we go further on the road to self-acceptance; and we know we have found

6. Merton, *Love and Living*, 35.

true self-acceptance when we can say to ourselves, "I wouldn't have it any other way."

When we expose society's false beliefs about beauty and worth, we are ready to see the hidden beauty within ourselves. We liberate ourselves to live authentically in the world as we quietly listen for the Truth—God. As we listen, God speaks a true word about ourselves, and our objections to our brokenness are wiped away one by one. We come to accept ourselves, willing and able to make peace with our brokenness. The peace allows us to live authentically: to unconditionally accept reality as experienced both in the self and in the world.

Nothing is more beautiful than a life lived to the fullest, no matter how horrible some of its circumstances may be, as my friends Lusseyran, Carretto, and Barfoot attest. When we live authentically, we are saying to the world, "This is who I am and am meant to be before God: no matter what you think of me, I will live as one true to myself and to God." When we embrace unwavering acceptance of life and self like a long-lost friend, not only do we know the truth of ourselves, but we accept it with joy. And when we allow this truth into our lives, we realize one of the most remarkable truths of all—our brokenness comes to us as a gift from God because it allows us to accept ourselves and others just as we are, in the fullness of our humanity.

FIVE

Discovering the Gift

The wonder of those long days of training, repeatedly pushing my body to the limit, led me closer to God and inspired me to go to a religious college to study physical education. My training logs had become a journal of my thoughts, prayers, and experiences. Not only had my body awakened to extraordinary new possibilities, but I was on the verge of coming to life intellectually.

My intellectual coming-of-age would be challenging, for my vocational education had not prepared me well for the rigors of college. But having won many physical battles, I knew how to fight. A burning desire overtook me as once again I set out to fulfill a dream. The dream wasn't so much to land that perfect job at the end of the college road as to make intellectual sense of my personal journey, the nature of physical movement, and God. I am happy to report that despite low test scores and an essay that would make any high-school English teacher cringe, I was accepted at Gordon College, a Christian liberal arts college north of Boston.

My professors enthusiastically greeted my project of understanding movement, God, and my disability. Not once did they criticize me for my goal of pursuing a degree in physical education. They encouraged me to pursue the answers I needed in a context of intellectual freedom, even though it would be nearly two years of struggle before the doors of my intellect would blow wide open and I would be able to think and write on the level expected of me.

My advisor, Dr. Peggy Hothem, took me under her wing and nurtured my intellectual and spiritual growth. She always believed in my ability to succeed. When I needed encouragement, she would remind me that my studies were a work in progress. At times she would say, "I see tremendous leadership potential." Like my mother, my dear professor never said "Can't."

Often I wanted to abandon my seat in the library that had become my daily home and be released from what seemed like my college prison. I knew Dr. Hothem would never let me leave without an explanation, though. So even when I wanted to march right into her office and blurt out, "That's it; I quit!" I could never come up with a proper explanation as to why I would leave. So I hung in there. When I felt like giving up, she'd sit and talk with me to find out why I was so frustrated. Usually it would be something like having hundreds of pages still left to read when I had been stuck in the library for what seemed like endless days. Right there in her office, we would have a word of prayer, and then back I'd go to my library home. Thanks to her encouragement, my intellectual self was born.

IN THE WILDERNESS

Gordon College is the home of the La Vida Center for Outdoor Education, whose wilderness program takes groups on wilderness adventures to teach lessons about faith and God. When I was a student, going on La Vida, as this program was called, was a requirement of all students. I could easily have asked to be excused from this requirement, but I chose not to. As a physical education major studying the value of such trips, I longed to have the same experiences as my classmates.

A wilderness trip that matched five disabled students with six able-bodied people was my brainchild. I met with school officials and convinced them to help me provide an adaptive program for the disabled students on campus. I then persuaded two other women with cerebral palsy, one blind man, and one man with a variety of visual and physical limitations to go out into the wilderness for some fun challenges such as rock climbing and canoeing. As I was scheming ways to sell the idea to the students and the administration, I had no idea of the impact the trip would have on my life. During our fourteen days in the wilderness, we would all discover strengths and weaknesses that we had never before suspected.

∾

The rain was falling on us hard, and we were cold and wet. We had to stop our canoe parade to wait for Carol and Hillary, who were lagging behind. Hillary, normally wheelchair bound because of her cerebral palsy, was sitting in a special chair welded to the front of the canoe. Her seat had a back that allowed her to support her torso. Carol, the strongest able-bodied member, was teamed up with Hillary, but Carol's strength and the special chair's support clearly were not enough. They were unable to keep up with the rest of us.

We were trying to keep the canoe teams together, but after three or four more stops in the pouring rain, we were losing heart. The waters of Saranac Lake in upstate New York were choppy. "If we don't keep moving, we will all get very cold," I said to my canoe mate, Tia. I didn't turn around and look, but I knew her face showed her agreement. I couldn't believe I was the one who had gotten us into this.

We could not repeatedly stop and wait in the stormy weather for Carol and Hillary. The previous day, when the sun had been shining, the rest of us used these breaks to put on more sunscreen or to look around us and chat about the beauty of the wilderness. But today the rain felt like sheets of cold water being poured over our heads, and this called for action.

Those of us in the five waiting canoes decided to have a group discussion about the situation. We paddled next to each other and hung onto the sides of each other's canoes as the water churned around us. Huddling together, we watched Carol and Hillary's progress. Carol paddled hard from the back end of her canoe as Hillary's paddle slapped the water awkwardly, preventing Carol from making much headway. Hillary's cerebral palsy was much more severe than mine. Both her arms and her legs were affected with not only weakness but also spasticity, and she had limited torso strength. The more Hillary tried to paddle, the more she slowed Carol down. The situation called for action, but who was willing to speak the truth?

As we got wetter and colder, I resolved to speak up. Eventually the two of them arrived at the side of our canoe, and Carol reached out and connected with us. As she did, I said something like, "Hillary, your paddling is not helping matters. It's slowing Carol down, and we are all wet and cold, and all we want to do is break camp as soon as possible so we can get warm. I am sorry if I am being harsh, but that's the truth, so sit back and relax. We're going to race through the rest of the lake now. We all have gifts and talents. Let us use ours now, and you will get your turn some other time."

We all broke apart from our circle, and away we went to conquer the second half of Saranac Lake. Our final destination was a portage marked out by our group leaders. They had taken us through this wilderness for a week, showing us the way. Then they had given us a map to follow along the lakes and portages and left us on our own for the final leg of our expedition. In a few hours we would meet them at the portage, and our journey would be complete.

As we began to increase our speed, Carol was out in front and probably colder than the rest of us. Hillary looked disappointed and upset. Suddenly Hillary's voice rang out through the cold and wet. Hillary's greatest gift was her voice. She began to sing for us, and her singing proved to be the most important thing that happened on that cold September afternoon. Her voice coming to us between the raindrops made us all reach deep inside ourselves for every last bit of strength we had. "Amazing grace, how sweet the sound . . ."

"Wow, there it is," my heart said. "Ah, that's just what we needed." When something is taken from us, something else is given. In my somewhat harsh redirection, Hillary found an opportunity, and, through the grace of God, she shared her gift of voice with us.

～

As Hillary discovered her gift, I would discover mine. My discovery would come during our rock-climbing expedition.

I looked at the rock's jagged edges and saw nowhere to put my hands and feet. I raised my feet one at a time, scraping each foot against the rock to see if it could catch an edge so I could start to climb. I tried and tried with no success. There simply was no way to get started.

Finding my way up the rock shouldn't have been a problem. After all, I had just scampered up the trail to the rock face mostly on my hands and knees, grabbing roots, rocks, tree stumps, or anything I could get my hands on to make my way. My cerebral palsy robs me of my balance, so crawling was a helpful technique on difficult terrains.

When I finally made it to the rock face, the leaders and the staff people of the La Vida program set us up for the climb. They adapted some of the climbs for the people who were more challenged than I am, but all of us were going to take part in a complete La Vida program, which meant that all of us would attempt to climb the rock. As I continued to scrape the rock face with my feet, trying to get started, Rich Obenschain, the program director, spotted my problem. He boosted me up to a ledge where I could get my footing and start climbing.

The boost made me angry because I hated my disabled body. For many years I had fought against my disability. I had worked hard to swing, skate, play sports, and even be a physical education major. There was just one thing I wanted, and that was to make my disability go away. I had spent my entire life up to that point—twenty-two years—trying to make myself as normal as possible.

The ledge on which I now stood provided me with plenty of nooks and crannies to help me propel myself forward. As I looked around, trying to scope out my next move, I couldn't help huddling close to the rock as if it were my best friend and whispering, "Lord, not on my strength, but your strength." Slowly, I began to grab whatever tiny little irregular pieces of rock I could find while thinking, "God is my stronghold and my crag."

While grasping all those lovable nooks and hugging the rock for dear life, I heard it. As I neared the top of the rock, someone watching my unique, broken, and disabled way of climbing shouted down toward me, "You are a blessing!" The words penetrated my ears and shot right through to my heart. A surge of energy ran through me. At that moment, love began to consume the hatred that had built up from years of ridicule as people stared and laughed at my disabled body. All the years of hating God's handiwork disappeared from every corner of my inner being. For the first time ever, God entered into the part of me that hated my disability. I realized again—as I had on the swings and on my ice skates, but now in a deeper way—God's thoughtful hand in creating me just as I am: broken, disabled, and yet whole.

Self-acceptance and its partner, self-love, flooded my being. After all those years of fighting, I came to know my broken body as a gift, a wonderful gift given to me by God. All the awkwardness, falls, struggle, and pain now spoke in a holy voice to the depths of my heart. God's love penetrated the years of accumulated self-hatred so that I could finally embrace my brokenness. Inner healing came to my soul. No longer fighting, I could begin to be myself in the world without concern for what others thought of my brokenness. No longer consumed by what I had to prove, I could begin to be who I was called to be: a woman of God who is broken and yet whole.

LETTING GOD INTO OUR PAIN

Those of us who struggle in pain must find something precious hiding in our brokenness. But how can we do this?

When tragedy strikes, God does not abandon us, but rather, God waits for us to respond. We cannot create any longing for God by our own power. God's grace mysteriously initiates our response by stirring up within us spiritual longings that enable us to reach out to experience God's love. We decide whether or not to act on these inner stirrings. When we begin to see the gift hiding in our tragedy, we also begin to know God's love in the midst of our pain.

The great Jewish philosopher Martin Buber told a Hasidic story showing the importance of our response to God:

"'Where is the dwelling of God?'

This was the question with which the Rabbi of Kotzk surprised a number of learned men who happened to be visiting him.

They laughed at him: 'What a thing to ask! Is not the whole world full of His glory?'

Then he answered his own question:

'God dwells wherever man lets Him in.'

This is the ultimate purpose: to let God in. But we can let Him in only where we really stand, where we live, where we live a true life."[1]

If we let God dwell in the midst of our suffering and pain, there God will be. By letting God in, we allow ourselves to experience God even in our suffering. By letting God in, we hear God speak through our suffering, bringing new life and transformation from within it.

Our culture, because it does not let God in, cannot know that God exists in what it considers worthless. The key for all of us who are broken is to let God in, hoping that others may see our humanity and need for love, and knowing that even in our brokenness, God gives his precious gift of love. When I let God in, my whole life becomes an offering.

But before we can let God in, we must accept ourselves. When the truth—what God would have us believe—about ourselves captivates us,

1. Martin Buber, *The Way of Man according to the Teachings of Hasidism* (Secaucus, NJ: Citadel, 1966) 41.

we are ready to let God in. Self-acceptance comes first because it allows us to open up our beings to a lasting union with God, so that God can dwell where life hurts us most. It is as if God says to us, "Here in your innermost self, at the bottom of your pain, you will find me."

When we invite God into the depths of our pain, God fills the emptiness that our brokenness has left in its wake. With God dwelling in our pain, the darkness is transformed into the light of God. It is changed into something precious; it becomes a gift. When this happens, our relationship with God enters a new dimension. When we pray, no longer do we come to God as if the Divine One is merely our provider. Instead, we come to God as to a partner who is ready, willing, and able to help us move forward in our journey to healing and wholeness.

SIX

Healing, Wholeness, and the Power of Christ

I HAD JUST BEGUN graduate studies at Temple University, and I was going to Woolworth's to buy an inexpensive desk lamp for my new apartment in Philadelphia. A woman on Market Street decided she wanted to pray for me, as she was praying for many near a busy bus stop.

To my eyes, this woman was either homeless or almost so. Her torn, dirty clothes gave her away. She wore a navy-blue knit hat, even though it was September, an unbuttoned red-and-blue-checked flannel shirt with about three cotton T-shirts underneath it, and a torn tan cotton skirt with a ruffled bottom. To complete her outfit, she had on ratty old Converse men's ankle-high canvas basketball sneakers, complete with men's tube socks.

I was just walking past the woman when she called out to me in a loud, holier-than-thou voice, "Have faith, and I will heal you! Do you believe in God?"

I said to myself, "Yes, I believe in God," and so her booming, confrontational voice hooked me in. I walked back toward the bench she was standing on, preaching to the crowds who were waiting for the bus or just enjoying the sunshine. As she stepped down from the bench, I wondered what was going to happen next. Here's how it went:

"Have faith and God will heal you," she said. "Come here and I will heal you." I decided to play along, knowing full well that God might have other plans for me. As she embraced me, I could feel the eyes of the crowd on me.

The woman invoked the Holy Spirit and said, "Now, my Father, heal this child. Heal this child and give her new strong legs. By her faith, let it be done to her."

I heard those words and I thought, "Here we go. Here comes the battle." She pushed me away from her bosom, expecting me to walk away leaping, and no doubt saying to herself, "God, I know that I have freed this child from Satan's grasp."

When I stumbled forward, obviously unhealed, the woman said to me, "You have no faith!"

The hair on the back of my neck stood up. She had not seen me ride a bike, swing up to the treetops, win a footrace, and triumph over all those who said, "She's not college material." All these things achieved through faith flashed through my mind as I now took center stage. With the power of my faith, I was ready to fight.

The crowd was enthralled. A few people climbed onto the bench where the woman had been preaching to watch the battle between the lame girl and the wannabe healer. I leaned in closely and looked up at the woman, as she was considerably taller than I was, and asked, "Were you there? Tell me if you were there. I want to know if you were there when God created the foundation of the world and decided my fate. I want to know if you were there when God spoke to Job in the whirlwind and asked him if Job himself was there when God created the heavens and the earth.[1] I want to know! Who are you to question my faith? You don't know the faith that I have. I will tell you the truth—it takes a lot more faith to walk around in the world as I do than it would take if I were somehow made perfect."

The woman's rotten teeth pointed down at me as she looked at me with mean eyes. I said, "If your ideas of faith are true, why are your teeth rotting in your mouth? Why has God not healed you of this? Maybe *you* lack faith!" I finished my speech and the crowd at the bus stop cheered and whistled. I turned and walked away.

If I had not come to know the gift hiding in my brokenness, per-haps I would have walked away sobbing. Perhaps I would have believed that God did not love me because I was not healed. Knowing that Jesus, throughout his ministry, healed brokenness, I might have asked: "Why isn't my brokenness healed today?"

Jesus does not turn away social outcasts like the poor, the lame, and the sick. One of my favorite healing stories is about a woman who was an outcast. She somehow found the courage to push through the crowd gathered around Jesus, in the hope of merely touching the fringe of his cloak. Here is her story as told in the Gospel according to Luke:

---

1. Job 38:4.

As he went, the crowds pressed in on him. Now there was a woman who had been suffering from hemorrhages for twelve years; and though she had spent all she had on physicians, no one could cure her. She came up behind him and touched the fringe of his clothes, and immediately her hemorrhage stopped. Then Jesus asked, "Who touched me?" When all denied it, Peter said, "Master, the crowds surround you and press in on you." But Jesus said, "Someone touched me; for I noticed that power had gone out from me." When the woman saw that she could not remain hidden, she came trembling; and falling down before him, she declared in the presence of all the people why she had touched him, and how she had been immediately healed. He said to her, "Daughter, your faith has made you well; go in peace."[2]

This story is a source of inspiration to me, not because the hemorrhaging stops when the woman touches Jesus's garment, but because of the faith underlying the entire healing encounter. In order for this woman to approach Jesus, she must first believe herself worthy of the healing Jesus has to offer. She must also believe that Jesus has the power and the willingness to heal her. This faith gives her the courage to push her way through the crowd. And indeed, Jesus shows compassion and love to this woman from the margins of society, though everyone else would have seen her as worthless. The woman is willing to act on behalf of her brokenness, and Jesus says at the end of the story that it is just this faithfulness that has restored her to wholeness.

We see her wholeness restored on the outside, but we must remember that there is more to healing than meets the eye, and it is difficult to discern from our lives what God intends. Much healing involves little or no restoration on the outside, but the person is being miraculously transformed inside. Whether healing is inside, outside, or both, it is based on faith—faith that we are worthy of being healed, faith that Jesus can and will heal us, faith to push past all obstacles between us and Jesus.

We can see and believe in inner healing only if we look at the situation with a mystical vision. Like Job, we weren't there when God created the foundation of the earth, so who are we to question God's wisdom now? If I were healed, would I have experienced the thrill, exhilaration, and beauty of that day when I crossed the finish line with four girls behind me? Would those two heavyset nuns have said such passionate and loving

2. Luke 8:42b–48 (NRSV).

prayers to God on my behalf? Would my experiences of swinging, skating, or riding a bike have lived on to give me such lasting hope? Would my life speak with the same voice? In the end, although it is a mystery, and we cannot begin to understand the wisdom of God, one thing is sure: we are all called to be who we are before God.

WHOLENESS

Saint Bernard of Clairvaux, a twelfth-century monastic reformer, said, "A wise man is one who savors all things as they really are."[3] In service to God, we courageously accept our lot in life, whatever it may be. This unconditional acceptance is an act of self-love that is easily misunderstood.

Several years ago while on a retreat, I commented on a New Testament story about a man who was disabled from birth. His friends carried him to the temple gate where he would beg. Day after day they did this, until one day when Peter and John, two disciples of Jesus, saw the man lying on the ground at the gate. The man asked Peter and John for money, and Peter replied,

"I have no silver or gold, but what I have I give you; in the name of Jesus Christ of Nazareth, stand up and walk. And he took him by the right hand and raised him up; and immediately his feet and ankles were made strong. Jumping up, he stood and began to walk, and he entered the temple with them, walking and leaping and praising God."[4]

I said, "I really feel for this man, disabled all his life—and now he must readjust everything. After all, he has only known disability and begging. If someone were to say to me, 'Come over here, stand in the middle of the room, and I will heal you,' I don't know whether I could."

The leader, Father Dan Berrigan, said, "I would like to take a different approach and say that the community would be supportive of this newly healed man and that he would adjust okay." A woman came up to me after the session and said, "I see that you don't want the fullness of what God has to offer you."

I felt like Satan's horns were growing out of my head. What was I trying to convey that got so badly misconstrued? Could my perception be that far off? Why would it be so difficult to be healed?

3. Quoted in Josef Pieper, *Living the Truth* (San Francisco: Ignatius, 1989) 108 and front cover.
4. Acts 3:6–8.

I struggled the entire night. Having read many religious works by Thomas Merton, Paul Tillich, Martin Buber, Abraham Joshua Heschel, and many others, I thought I understood what faith was about. I considered myself a devout lover of God, and I believed I was faithfully living out God's call to me. At the time of this retreat, I was considering whether or not to go to divinity school in preparation for priesthood in the Episcopal Church. Should I be seeking healing? Had my faith truly missed the mark? And if my faith was not off target, then what was it about not being healed that was so alarming to Father Dan and the others?

In times like this, prayer is my only refuge. The idea that I was not seeking the fullness of what God had to offer me was most disturbing. So I prayed nearly the entire night, and when morning came, I slipped off into the retreat grounds to pray still more as all the others were eating breakfast. I opened myself up and left my torment in God's holy hands.

As everyone else formed small groups to discuss the opening topic of the morning, my friend Frances Innes-Mitchell and I remained in a corner of the spacious modern room of the convent where the retreat was held. I couldn't get into a small group. I needed to just be. Frances understood, so we sat quietly together.

Father Dan came by and greeted us as he sipped his morning coffee. Frances, who also has cerebral palsy, asked Father Dan a question. He bent down to hear, and she repeated: "Do you think some people have a vocation to be disabled?"

As soon as her question was out, words poured forth from my depths. Father Dan stared off into space as he listened, deep in thought. As I neared the end of what I had to say, he suddenly stopped me midsentence and stood straight up as if he had received an electric shock. "Would you mind sharing that with the rest of the group?" he asked.

Remembering my prayers of the morning, I agreed. Father Dan called out to the entire retreat group, "Something very unusual is coming from this corner of the room." Everyone turned to listen.

As I spoke, my spasticity made my legs kick out straight, and my hair felt like it was standing on end. God was clearly evident—and so was my disability. I said: "Someone may look at me and ask, 'Where is the miracle? Where is the healing? Where is God?' To them I say, my brokenness is one of the ways God speaks to me, and it is one of the ways I know God. Yes, there are times when pain and suffering are great, and we need to ask for it to be removed; but when brokenness stays, it is for a reason, and sometimes that reason opens the way for us to know God."

A man came up to me after my impassioned speech and said, "As you spoke, I realized these are not the words of someone who is broken, but someone who is whole!" My entire healing journey was in that speech. My perspective on my brokenness and its meaning in my life had changed so profoundly over the years that now, after I had lived with my disability for thirty-some years, it had been mysteriously and miraculously transformed from a tragedy into a gift given to me by God. The healing that began on the rock face nine years earlier now became even more real to me, as my self-hatred over my brokenness continued to be transformed by the love of God.

The gift of God hiding in brokenness did not come to me all at once, but in stages. Over the years, I developed an identity of wholeness. This identity comes to us when we have traveled a long way on the healing journey and find ourselves transforming suffering almost effortlessly. The suffering handed to us by chance becomes a part of ourselves that we accept as if it came from the hand of God. We know that our brokenness is not only the harbinger of pain but also a messenger of God's love. And in God's words of love, we find the secret to our true identity: we are loved even though we are broken.

Wholeness lives within and behind brokenness. Our true identity in God can be fully known only through a religious encounter in which God touches us in our pain. When God is encountered in brokenness, the hidden goodness and meaning of brokenness are unveiled. Through the unveiling, God interacts with the suffering self and transforms it: where we once knew ourselves as broken, we now know ourselves as whole. The unveiling allows all of us to know our true humanity before God while we exclaim together, "I am made whole by the love of God!" Our intimate encounter with God gives us the opportunity to know ourselves as whole even though we are broken.

But how can someone be broken and yet whole? Our wholeness is a gift from God. Where we are fractured, God envelops our brokenness with God's own undeniable wholeness. As we step out in faith in spite of our brokenness and let God more deeply into our inner world, we become more and more aware that God is seeping through the cracks of what is hurting us the most. God continually, over and over again, fills the void caused by our fractured lives. The more we learn to look, the more we see God's light, love, and healing peeking through the crevices where our lives are most disturbed. What else can we do when we discover this truth but simply say thank you as we accept our lot as a gift? When we truly understand God's wholeness, the peace and transformation it brings are remarkable. I am sure that is what kept Carlo Carretto in the Sahara, enabled Jacques Lusseyran to survive Buchenwald, and allowed Edith Barfoot to give such a powerful testimony when wracked with so much pain.

My God is the God of Abraham, Isaac, and Jacob, the God of both Christianity and Judaism. I seek to be inclusive of my Jewish friends. I also want to preserve the fact that I am called as a Christian to preserve my individuality and testify to the truth of what I believe, and I believe that Jesus gives us this gift of wholeness that hides mysteriously in our brokenness. If you find the idea of Jesus's giving us wholeness hard to swallow, at least understand this before you continue reading: Jesus Christ is the way I have intimacy with God. Union with God is the end result that we all seek. If you are not a Christian, reflect on what it means to obtain intimacy with God in terms of your own conception of faith, and translate what I am about to say into words that fit with your beliefs. What is most important here is what your inner being experiences as faith leading you to intimacy with God.

～

God moves toward union with humanity, first through creating the world and then through making a covenant with Abraham and his descendants, the people of Israel. Eventually (so Christians believe) God becomes human in the birth of Jesus. Though fully divine as well as fully human, Jesus lives and dies as one of us. He teaches the ignorant and the learned, comforts the poor and the outcast, and heals the disabled and the sick. After a short ministry, Jesus is crucified. But then, to the bewilderment of his followers, he appears to them again. He has risen from the dead!

The New Testament's primary message is that God loves us, God has become one of us, and God will remain with us forever. Through Jesus, God's relationship to humanity is transformed. Now intimacy with God is made available to us by way of faith in Jesus Christ.

Jesus opens up to us a whole new view of reality. As one who suffered deeply, he affirms the possibility for us to experience wholeness even in our brokenness. The Hebrew prophet Isaiah expresses this beautifully:

> He was despised and rejected by others;
> a man of suffering and acquainted with infirmity;
> and as one from whom others hide their faces
> he was despised, and we held him of no account.
> Surely he has borne our infirmities
> and carried our diseases;
> yet we accounted him stricken,
> struck down by God, and afflicted.
> But he was wounded for our transgressions,
> crushed for our iniquities;
> upon him was the punishment that made us whole,
> and by his bruises we are healed.[5]

Wholeness is a gift truly made real through Jesus Christ. When Jesus died and rose again, he unified brokenness and all the other tragedies of the world with the fullness of God. The power that transformed Jesus's brokenness into resurrection can transform our brokenness into new life. Through faith in Jesus Christ, we can experience wholeness even in our brokenness, because Christ's sacrifice gives us access to the transformative power of intimacy with God.

I believe that divine healing power comes through Christ. You may believe it comes from another source. Regardless of its source, faith is required to access it. I cannot explain the transformative powers of other faiths because Christianity is my faith, and I know no other power than that which Christ gives me. If you live by another faith, you can seek intimacy with Divine One or the Ultimate through that faith according to your own understanding.

For Christians, intimacy with God comes in a new way since the resurrection. The resurrected Christ, one with God the Father and the Holy Spirit, permeates the entire universe as an invisible reality. Our brokenness is held within this larger and invisible reality of Christ's wholeness. At the same time, God dwells in our brokenness, so we can experience it no longer as brokenness but as wholeness that comes to us as a gift from our union with God.

---

5. Isaiah 53:3–5 (NRSV).

If God dwells in our fractured beings and bodies, we are people to whom healing has come. As divine love touches the jagged edges of our brokenness, God's complete and everlasting wholeness expresses itself in our lives. God's light penetrates through the darkness, and love and goodness greatly abound. Our healing is hidden to those who cannot look into the depths of reality with a spiritual eye, but it is true just the same.

I experienced the wholeness that comes to us through Christ when I spoke up while on retreat with Dan Berrigan. However, I would sense this wholeness even more fully a few years later while doing my field placement as part of my seminary education at the University of Chicago Divinity School. Required to participate in church-related duties and liturgical functions with my broken body, I was forced to look deeply into the meaning of wholeness as it is given to us by God. It took years for me to gain the courage to partake in these sacred acts. My understanding of wholeness would continue to grow as God persistently called me to serve the church.

WHOLENESS IN ACTION

The stained-glass windows at the front of Emmanuel Parish Episcopal Church show Jesus standing in dazzling white apparel with his arms opened wide as if to reach out and hold me. As a young child I knew God loved me, not because we went to church very often, but because that picture of Jesus helped me through my struggles. So one day, cuddled up to my mother's side as someone read Psalm 107 out of the *Book of Common Prayer* ("The LORD changed rivers into deserts, / and water-springs into thirsty ground . . .").[6] I said to myself, "Someday I am going to learn how to do that." Someday, I meant, I am going to learn how to stand up in front of a church and read the psalms.

My return to the University of Chicago for my second year in the Master of Divinity program was nothing short of a miracle. My route took me through the scenic roads of Vermont to I-90, where the road bears either to the left toward Boston or to the right toward Buffalo and on to Chicago. Perplexed, I turned toward Boston, saying to myself, "You don't want to go to Chicago. It only means very difficult things."

6. *The Book of Common Prayer* (New York: Oxford University Press, 1979) 748.

After a few miles I said to myself, "You don't want to go toward Boston. It only means the same old things. You want more for your life." So I turned around.

Now traveling toward Buffalo, I began to consider all the difficult things I would have to do this year, such as being a chalice minister (walking while carrying a full cup of wine) and preaching. "No, no, no, you don't want this at all," I thought, pounding my fist on the steering wheel. I turned around again. But as I traveled back toward Boston I thought, "What are you going back to? You're chasing your same old life."

Finally, after circling for an hour, I stopped at a hotel, hoping to use a clean restroom. There was no public restroom, but there was a public pay phone. Maybe someone could help me stop circling the wagons and get on with the ride.

The first few people I called weren't home. I then reached a close friend who said, "Stop driving. Don't go anywhere until you are sure you know where you want to go, and then go there and don't look back."

"But, but—" I replied, in deep distress.

"No buts," she said, asking me to call her later to tell her what state I was in.

I got back in my car and waited and waited. I waited some more. Then I heard the voice that I sometimes have the courage to name God. It said, "Go, go, you must go . . ."

Fear of the physical movement required to perform my duties as a seminarian (one who is training for the priesthood) is what had me circling on the interstate. The physicality of ministry is easy to miss if you are not looking for it. We are so used to it that we don't realize how much is involved. Liturgical objects and actions are used to touch the senses in the hope of bringing an experience of the divine. Holy elements are involved: bread, wine, books, movement, special clothing, and flaming candles, to name a few. It is important that they be handled with care. For many, consecrated communion wine is Jesus himself in the chalice. Spilling the wine spells disaster.

I almost quit my field education over fear of spilling the communion wine. As a chalice minister, I would carry a cup of wine to the people gathered at the altar during communion. Usually there is an altar rail around the area where people kneel to receive communion. Saint Paul and the Redeemer Church, where I did my field placement, has no altar rail. As a church with a modern focus, it has installed a temporary altar closer to the congregation that consists of a five-by-fifteen-foot half-circle. Because the altar is level with the congregation, it is easier for older and disabled people to come and receive communion. People can stand, kneel, or sit as they receive the bread and wine.

This half-circle with no altar rail and people standing, kneeling, or sitting worried me. When you are disabled, things like icy sidewalks and tile floors with cracks are causes for concern; oftentimes, everyday situations require systematic planning much like that a skilled mountain climber makes before scaling a cliff. So, long before I ever had to hold the sacred cup, I examined all the movements necessary to complete the task. I would watch others giving people the wine and think, "It's down and toward the lips with the chalice and then, okay, bend up, pray that you don't fall. Now careful, and on to the next person."

My most graphic fear, which played over and over in my mind like a recurring nightmare, was that I would topple over with the chalice, hear it clang to the linoleum floor, and see a puddle of wine trickling down the middle of the aisle between the pews. The puddle of Jesus (because Jesus, in the minds of many Episcopalians, would be present in the consecrated wine) would stay there waiting to be mopped up by some mortified parishioner. Trust me, it would not be a good thing for me to fall headlong, spewing the blood of Christ on the floor or in someone's face.

I prayed about this fear the night before I had to give church members the sacred wine for the first time. I fall nearly every day. A muscle spasm can hurl me to the ground in seconds flat. When this happens, my legs just give way. It is as if they protest, "That's it, I am not going to hold you up anymore," and down I go. I'm used to falling, but I did not want to fall in such a sacred situation. Not only would a fall disturb the worship of hundreds of people, but it might also offend God. These are the thoughts that were strangling the life out of me the night before my first stint as chalice minister.

Sunday, I went to the 8:00 a.m. service so that I could discuss my anxieties with my teaching pastor, Reverend Jim Steen, before being chalice minister at 10:00. I wanted to devise an escape route if carrying the sacred cup proved to be too much for me. I never got the chance. As I walked into the church building, Reverend Steen raced over to me and said, "Did someone call you?"

"No," I said as my anxiety skyrocketed.

"The deacon isn't here today. Would you mind being chalice minister?" he asked.

The clock read 7:56. I said, "Yes, I will do it," knowing that a detailed discussion of my crisis was out of the question. Anxiety filled me. You know the kind of anxiety—when your stomach feels like it's going to explode, your head feels like it's severed from your body (though you can feel it pounding away at a distance), and all your legs want to do is run away. God was pushing me to my limits.

Shortly after the sermon, I took my place at the altar. I suddenly saw that the pastor had filled the cup to the brim. In my alarmed state, I thought, "How am I going to carry this wine from person to person along this altar if it's so full?" *Full, full, full!* my mind screamed, as I looked down into the wine. The first rule if you're going to pour me a drink is, you have to leave room. But there was no room in this chalice for any of the wine to slosh from side to side. So, problem solver that I am, my first thought was, *I* have to make room!

Traditionally the chalice minister takes a sip of wine before all the others drink. So, I thought, drink it down. I turned my back to the parishioners so they couldn't see my swollen cheeks filled with wine. I knew I couldn't take a second "sip" or my pastor might think I had a drinking problem. My big swig went down the hatch, and the level in the chalice went down. Now that the cup was safe for me to walk with, I gave each person gathered around the altar a sip of wine.

After the first group is done, the chalice bearer walks back to the starting place while the next group gets the bread. On that first journey back, you could see wine droplets splashing around the chalice as if a storm had hit. Fortunately, every drop was spared the fate of hitting the floor, although one parishioner saw the sloshing wine and looked frightened at what might happen next. The eight and ten o'clock services both went fine; there were no catastrophes.

Carrying the chalice, dressing in sacred clothes, and reading prayers, one becomes a liturgical presence. One's body expresses something sacred. Each body has a voice that speaks through its actions, manner, and presence. I first noticed this when Zarina O'Hagin, our deacon, reads the gospel. She joins the gospel procession smiling and beaming with the love of Christ. She holds the gospel book up high with love illuminating her face and announces, "The Holy Gospel of our Lord Jesus Christ!" She moves out into the congregation with grace and poise as if to say, This is the gospel that the Lord has given to us. Her manner says to everyone, This is a gospel of joy, new life, and resurrection.

She would not have to say a word; it is all so simple to understand when she uses her body. As I watched Zarina week after week, I realized that our physical movements while facing the congregation are a means of sacred expression. I became concerned with my own presence. If I lurch up the aisle with a flaming candle, some may see my distorted movement as ugly or unbecoming for such a sacred context. I began to ask myself questions about my broken body and its meaning for ministry. What does my body say to others? Does it speak a word of beauty, love, and redemption, or does it merely communicate brokenness? Is it right for me to teeter with communion cups of wine? Is my body as a sacred presence offensive to anyone? The answers to these questions came near the end of my field placement when I truly learned the meaning of being a sacred presence, as expressed in my unique embodiment as a woman with a disability.

"The blood of Christ, the cup of salvation," I say as I tip the cup toward Mrs. Jones's lips. Her eyes look reverently at me, and as she takes the cup, I see my reflection in the silver chalice. In the communion cup, my garment, an alb, looks like Christ's dazzling white garment in the stained-glass window of my home church. I remember again what I said as a child: "Someday I am going to learn how to do that."

More people come to the altar. The reverent looks continue. Taking the utmost care not to fall, concentrating ever so carefully just as I did in front of all those doctors at Children's Hospital, seeking to walk perfectly for God, I continue to see my reflection in the communion cup. "The blood of Christ, the cup of salvation," I murmur.

Over and over I see the reflection of my body, and my being says, "This is my broken body, and it serves this church. My body shows people what we do with brokenness in the church. Here in this cup is new life, and here is my body, expressing the truth of what this new life means!" As the people drink from the cup, I realize what my body is expressing to the congregation and all the people I serve: that Jesus gives us the power to know wholeness even in our brokenness. It is as if Jesus handed me the communion cup and said to me, "Serve my church."

Years later, Carlo Carretto would teach me that in the act of communion, we come to know the wholeness of God that is given to us as a gift.

As Carretto was lying on a mat, trying to deal with the pain of his newly disabled leg, he began to meditate on the meaning of the Eucharist. He was thinking and praying about what Jesus actually does in the thin wafer that, he believed, becomes Jesus, when a wonderful truth came to him. Carretto writes:

"In the Eucharist Jesus is immobilized not in one leg only, but both, and in his hands as well. He is reduced to a little piece of white bread. The world needs him so much and yet he doesn't speak. We need him so much and he doesn't move!"[7]

In the Eucharist, Christ imitates our brokenness as he gives us the power to know wholeness, even when we are broken. And when the Eucharist is in us, Christ acts through us. Knowing wholeness within ourselves, we are able to offer wholeness to the world through our experiences. We can express the truth that we are made whole by the love of God. A famous prayer attributed to Saint Teresa of Avila shows how we are Christ's body here on earth:

> Christ has no body now, but yours.
> No hands, no feet on earth, but yours.
> Yours are the eyes through which Christ looks compassion into
> the world.
> Yours are the feet with which Christ walks to do good.
> Yours are the hands with which Christ blesses the world.

Now that we have come to know wholeness within ourselves as it is given to us through Christ, we are obliged to give that same wholeness to the world. So as Christ is embodied in our hands, in our feet, and through our eyes, we go into the world putting wholeness into action.

How does Christ move through our imperfect and broken bodies to express his love and goodness to the world? When our actions are recognized as having an origin in God, our culture's lies about brokenness disintegrate into nothing. Those who perceive reality with a spiritual eye recognize us as truly whole, not lacking anything, for the mysterious wholeness of God's love (which to me is Christ) permeates our entire being. How holy is God upon the earth! Real beauty, dignity, self-

---

7. Carlo Carretto, *Letters from the Desert*, trans. Rose Mary Hancock (Maryknoll, NY: Orbis, 2002) 119.

acceptance, and truth come through the intimate touch of God, holding us and making us whole even in our brokenness, so that we in turn can share that wholeness with the world. And as we share that wholeness, we lead others to the same transformation we have been given through the glory of God. Amen.

THE WORD MY BODY SPEAKS

My body has a voice, and the word it speaks is love.

So do I choose life no matter what it will bring me? My answer is yes, and ironically the anoxia that hit my brain was indeed a tragedy, but through faith, hope, and love, new possibilities came to life and brought me into loving intimacy with God. If we look at our brokenness through the eyes of faith, as Lusseyran, Carretto, and Barfoot attest, we find God's love dwelling in our tragic circumstances. Over and over again—through the swing, the ripples in the pool, my bike, the basketball game, rock climbing—God has revealed this to be true, because God continually speaks a word of love through my awkward and teetering gait.

The tragic event of our brokenness takes on new meaning when the hidden goodness living inside it is made real to us. And as we struggle with brokenness, we can find new meaning in ourselves through understanding the reality of concealed wholeness. Because God lives in our brokenness, we are people of true worth.

God intended something beautiful in my brokenness, although it may remain hidden to those who cannot see with a mystical vision. My broken body may have little worth to our culture, but it has remarkable value to God. My brokenness gives me insight into true reality, and it is a window into my being. Through it I've found the wellspring of God's love that lives deep in my soul and my own hidden wholeness.

We discover this hidden wholeness when God touches us, and we come to know the truth of ourselves as we continue to live with God. Finding wholeness is an inner experience hidden deep within our union with God. It is a journey from self-hatred to self-acceptance. And it is a gift from God.

God's gift giving never leaves us. Although the gift may be hidden, it is with us just the same. To discover it, we must enter an inner world where God dwells with us. In this place, the divine presence touches our

deepest need for love. Encountering God moves us beyond our brokenness to a world of hidden goodness.

I believe that God's love is in our brokenness, constantly speaking a
word of love. Let there be no doubt: God has been speaking this word of
love in my brokenness throughout my life. My hope is that you too can
discover that love and experience its awesome healing power. Now that
you have read these pages, I hope you too can say, "It is wonderful that
I exist just as I am, broken and yet whole." For truly a word is spoken
through your brokenness, and the word is *love*.

www.ingramcontent.com/pod-product-compliance
Lightning Source LLC
Chambersburg PA
CBHW030843090426
42737CB00009B/1096